THE SYNOPSIS OF MEDICINE

PARAMEDICAL & NURSING STUDENTS

DR S SINGH

Copyright © Dr S Singh
All Rights Reserved.

ISBN 978-1-64951-021-1

This book has been published with all efforts taken to make the material error-free after the consent of the author. However, the author and the publisher do not assume and hereby disclaim any liability to any party for any loss, damage, or disruption caused by errors or omissions, whether such errors or omissions result from negligence, accident, or any other cause.

While every effort has been made to avoid any mistake or omission, this publication is being sold on the condition and understanding that neither the author nor the publishers or printers would be liable in any manner to any person by reason of any mistake or omission in this publication or for any action taken or omitted to be taken or advice rendered or accepted on the basis of this work. For any defect in printing or binding the publishers will be liable only to replace the defective copy by another copy of this work then available.

The book is dedicated to my Father... "To the world you may be one person, but to me you are the world"

Contents

Foreword — vii

Preface — ix

Acknowledgements — xi

1. Fever — 1
2. Polyuria — 6
3. Heart Disease — 7
4. Burns — 9
5. Vomiting — 14
6. Diarrhoea — 18
7. Jaundice — 22
8. Pneumonia — 27
9. Ascites — 33
10. Hepatitis — 43
11. Malaria — 47
12. Typhoid Fever — 56
13. Acquired Immunodeficiency Syndrome (aids) — 59
14. Pleural Effusion — 66
15. Tuberculosis — 69
16. Dyspnea, asphyxia & Hypoxia — 76
17. Cynosis — 84
18. Hypertension — 86
19. Cardiac Monitor — 95
20. Hemiplegia & Paraplegia — 98
21. Paralysis & Parkinson Disease — 102
22. Coma — 110
23. Diabetes Mellitus — 115
24. Addison`s Disease & Hypothyroidism — 119
25. Asthma — 127
26. Gastroenteritis — 140
27. Meningitis — 145
28. Renal Colic & Hypoglycemia — 154
29. Poison — 163

Foreword

Rights reserved. No parts of this publication may be reproduced, stored in a retrieval system, or transmitted, in any form or by any means, electronic, mechanical, photocopying, recording, or otherwise, without the prior permission of the author.

© *Dr S Singh*
Title - SYNOPSIS OF MEDICINE
FOR NURSING & OT TECHNICIAN
Author- Dr S Singh

Preface

The broad goal of the book on Medicine is to provide knowledge, skills and behavioral attribute that may enable the students & professionals of Nursing, Operation theatre technicians & Allied Healthcare workers to function effectively in a community setting and to help them understand the basic principle of history taking and clinical examinations.. The book explains about acute medical emergencies like acute myocardial infarction, acute pulmonary oedema, acute anaphylactic and hypovolumic shock, status asthmaticus, hyperpyrexia, , gastro-intestinal bleeding, diabetic coma, electric shock, drowning, snake bites, common poisoning etc. We are entering into an amazing era of knowledge and this book comprehend the basic principles involved in the management of the patient and initiate first line management.

Acknowledgements

I must extend my deepest gratitude to the all my colleagues, all of whom gave so freely of their time. Their suggestions and critical readings of the manuscript were invaluable. Any errors or lapses of judgment that remain are entirely my responsibility

THE SYNOPSIS OF MEDICINE

FOR

NURSING & OT TECHNICIAN

By Dr. S Singh

CHAPTER ONE

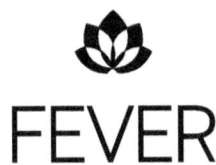

FEVER

Cyanosis is the appearance of a blue or purple coloration of the skin or mucous membranes due to the tissues near the skin surface being low on oxygen. The onset of cyanosis is 2.5g/dL of deoxyhemoglobin. The bluish color is more readily apparent in those with high hemoglobin counts than it is ith those with anemia. Also, the bluer color is more difficult to detect on deeply pigmented skin. When signs of cyanosis first appear, such as on the lips or fingers, intervention should be made within 3–5 minutes because a severe hypoxia or severe circulatory failure has induced thecyanosis.

The name *cyanosis*, literally means "the blue disease" or "the blue condition". It is derived from the color cyan, which comes from *kyanos*, the Greek word for blue.

Human blood is always a shade of red, and the more oxygenated the blood the brighter the shade of red. The more deoxygenated the blood, the darker red it is within the blood vessels, and the more bluish it appears on the skin. This color shift occurs because the optical properties of skin shift the darker red colors towards the bluer. (Some colors are refracted and absorbed more than others.) A similar phenomenon makes the sky appearblue.

Definition

Cyanosis is defined as a bluish discoloration, especially of the skin and mucous membranes due to excessive concentration of deoxyhemoglobin in the blood.

Differential diagnosis

Cyanosis is divided in to two main types: central (around the core and lips) and peripheral (only the extremities are affected). Cyanosis can occur in the fingers, including underneath the fingernails, as well as other extremities (called peripheral cyanosis), or in the lips and tongue (central cyanosis).

Central cyanosis

Central cyanosis is often due to a circulatory or ventilatory problem that leads to poor blood oxygenation in the lungs. It develops when arterial saturation of blood with oxygen is ≤85%. Cyanosis may not be detected until saturation is 75% in dark-skinned individuals.

Acute cyanosis can be a result of asphyxiation or choking, and is one of the surest signs that respiration is being blocked.

Causes
Central NervousSystem:

Intracranialhemorrhage
Cerebralanoxia
Drug overdose (e.g.Heroin)
RespiratorySystem:
Bronchiolitis
Bronchospasm (e.g.Asthma)
Lungdisease

Pulmonary embolism
Hypoventilation
COPD (emphysema and chronic bronchitis)
Cardiac Disorders:
>Congenital heart disease (e.g. Tetralogy of Fallot, right to left shunts in heart or great vessels)
Heart failure
Heart valve disease
Myocardial infarction
Blood:
Methemoglobinemia
Polycythemia
Others:

High altitude
Hypothermia
>Congenital cyanosis (HbM Boston) arises from a mutation in the α-codon which results in a change of primary sequence, H→
Y. Tyrosine stabilizes the Fe (III) form (oxyhemoglobin) creating a permanent T-state of Hb.
Obstructive sleep apnea
Peripheral cyanosis

Peripheral cyanosis is the blue tint in fingers or extremities, due to inadequate circulation. The blood reaching the extremities is not oxygen rich and when viewed through the skin a combination of factors can lead to the appearance of a blue color. All factors contributing to central cyanosis can also cause peripheral symptoms to appear, however peripheral cyanosis can be observed without there being heart or lung failures. Small blood vessels may be restricted and can be treated by increasing the normal oxygenation level of the blood.

Causes

All common causes of central cyanosis
Arterial obstruction
Cold exposure (due to vasoconstriction)
Raynaud's phenomenon (vasoconstriction)
Reduced cardiac output (e.g. heart failure, hypovolemia)
Vasoconstriction
Venous obstruction (e.g. deep vein thrombosis)
Differential cyanosis

Differential cyanosis is the bluish coloration of the lower but not the upper extremity and the head. This is seen in patients with a patent ductus arteriosus. Patients with a large ductus develop progressive pulmonary vascular disease, and pressure overload of the right ventricle occurs. As soon as pulmonary pressure exceeds aortic pressure, shunt reversal (right-to-left shunt) occurs. The upper extremity remains pink because the brachiocephalic trunk, left common carotid trunk and the left subclavian trunk is given off proximal to the PDA.

FEVER -HISTORY TAKING AND SYMPTOMALOGY

Fever (also known as pyrexia or hyperthermia is a common medical sign which is characterized by an elevation of temperature above the normal range that is 36.5–37.5 °C (98–100 °F) due to an increase in the body temperature regulatory set-point. This increase in set-point triggers increased muscle tone and shivering.

As a person's temperature increases, there is, a feeling of cold despite an increase in body temperature. Once the new temperature is reached, there is a feeling of warmth. A fever can be caused by many different conditions ranging from benign to potentially serious. Except for very high temperatures, treatment to reduce fever is often not necessary; however, antipyretic medications can be effective at lowering the temperature, which may improve the affected person's comfort.

Definition

Normal body temperatures vary depending on many factors, including age, sex, time of day, ambient temperature, activity level, and more. A raised temperature is not always a fever.

For example, the temperature of a healthy person rises when he or she exercises, but this is not considered a fever, as the set-point is normal.

Types

The pattern of temperature changes may occasionally hint at the diagnosis:

Continuous fever: Temperature remains above normal throughout the day and does not fluctuate more than 1 °C in 24 hours, *e.g.* lobar pneumonia, typhoid, urinary tract infection, brucellosis, or typhus. Typhoid fever may show a specific fever pattern, with a slow stepwise increase and a high plateau. (Drops due to fever-reducing drugs are excluded.)

Intermittent fever: The temperature elevation is present only for a certain period, later cycling back to normal, *e.g.* malaria, kala-azar, pyemias, or septicemia. Following are its types

Quotidian fever, with a periodicity of 24 hours, typical of Malaria

Tertian fever (48-hour periodicity), typical of Malaria

Quartan fever (72-hour periodicity), typical of *Plasmodium malaria*).

Remittent fever: Temperature remains above normal throughout the day and fluctuates more than 1 °C in 24 hours, *e.g.*, infective endocarditis.

Pel-Ebstein fever: A specific kind of fever associated with Hodgkin's lymphoma, is high for one week and low for the next week and so on. However, there is some debate as to whether this pattern truly exists

Hyperpyrexia

Hyperpyrexia is a fever with an extreme elevation of body temperature greater than or equal to 41.5 °C (106.7 °F). Such a high temperature is considered a medical emergency as it may indicate a serious underlying condition or lead to significant side effects. The most common cause is an intracranial haemorrhage and Other possible causes include sepsis, Kawasaki syndrome neuroleptic malignant syndrome, drug effects, serotonin syndrome, and thyroid storm. Infections are the most common cause of fevers, however as the temperature rises other causes become more common Infections commonly associated with hyperpyrexia include: roseola, rubeola and enteroviral infections Immediate aggressive cooling to less than 38.9 °C (102.0 °F) have been found to improve survival. Hyperpyrexia differs from hyperthermia in that in hyperpyrexia the body's temperature regulation mechanism sets the body temperature above the normal temperature, then generates heat to achieve this temperature, while in hyperthermia the body temperature rises above its set point.

Hyperthermia

Hyperthermia is an example of a high temperature that is not a fever. It occurs from several causes including heatstroke, neuroleptic malignant syndrome, malignant hyperthermia, stimulants such as amphetamines and cocaine, idiosyncratic drug reactions, and serotonin syndrome.

Signs and symptoms

A fever is usually accompanied by sickness behaviour, which consists of lethargy, depression, anorexia, sleepiness, hyperalgesia, and the inability to concentrate.

Differential diagnosis

Fever is a common symptom of many medical conditions:

Infectious disease, *e.g.*, influenza, HIV, malaria, or gastroenteritis

Various skin inflammations, *e.g.*, boils, or abscess

Immunological diseases, *e.g.*, lupus erythematosus, inflammatory bowel diseases

Tissue destruction, which can occur in hemolysis, surgery, infarction, etc.

Reaction to incompatible blood products

Cancers, most commonly kidney cancer and leukemia and lymphomas

Metabolic disorders, *e.g.*, gout or porphyria

Thrombo-embolic processes, *e.g.*, pulmonary embolism or deep venous thrombosis

Persistent fever that cannot be explained after repeated routine clinical inquiries is called fever of unknown origin.

Pathophysiology

Temperature is ultimately regulated in the hypothalamus. A trigger of the fever, called a pyrogen, causes a release of prostaglandin E2 (PGE2). PGE2 then, in turn, acts on the hypothalamus, which generates a systemic response back to the rest of the body, causing heat-creating effects to match a new temperature level.

In many respects, the hypothalamus works like a thermostat When the set point is raised, the body increases its temperature through both active generations of heat and retaining heat. Vasoconstriction both reduces heat loss through the skin and causes the person to feel cold. If these measures are insufficient to make the blood temperature in the brain match the new setting in the hypothalamus, then shivering begins to use muscle movements to produce more heat. When the fever stops, and the hypothalamic setting is set lower; the reverse of these processes (vasodilation, end of shivering and non-shivering heat production) and sweating are used to cool the body to the new, lower setting.

This contrasts with hyperthermia, in which the normal setting remains, and the body overheats through undesirable retention of excess heat or over-production of

heat. Hyperthermia is usually the result of an excessively hot environment (heat stroke) or an adverse reaction to drugs. Fever can be differentiated from hyperthermia by the circumstances surrounding it and its response to antipyretic medications.

Pyrogens

A pyrogen is a substance that induces fever. These can be either internal (endogenous) or external(exogenous) to the body. The bacterial substance lipopolysaccharide (LPS), present in the cell wall of some bacteria, is an example of an exogenous pyrogen.

Pyrogenicity can vary: In extreme examples, some bacterial pyrogens known

as superantigens can cause rapid and dangerous fevers. De-pyrogenation may be achieved through filtration, distillation, chromatography, or inactivation.

Research has demonstrated that fever has several important functions in the healing process:

Increased mobility of leukocytes

Enhanced leukocytes phagocytosis

Endotoxin effects decreased

Increased proliferation of T cells

Management

Fever should not necessarily be treated. Most people recover without specific medical attention Although it is unpleasant, fever rarely rises to a dangerous level even if untreated. Damage to the brain generally does not occur until temperatures reach 42 °C (107.6 °F),

and it is rare for an untreated fever to exceed 105 °F (41 °C). In general, people are advised to keep adequately hydrated, as the most significant risk of complications is dehydration.

Water is generally used for this purpose.

The use of a fan or air conditioning may somewhat reduce the temperature and increase comfort. If the temperature reaches an extremely high level of hyperpyrexia, aggressive cooling is required.

Medications

The antipyretic ibuprofen is effective in reducing fevers in children. it is more effective

than acetaminophen (paracetamol) in children. Ibuprofen and acetaminophen may be safely used together in children with fevers.

Etymology

Pyrexia is derived from the Greek word *pyretos* meaning *fire*. Febrile is from the Latin word *febris*, meaning *fever*, and archaically known as *ague*.

CHAPTER TWO

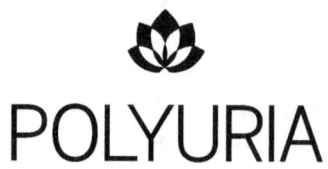

POLYURIA

Polyuria   -History taking and symptomatology

Polyuria is a condition usually defined as excessive or abnormally large production or passage of urine (at least 3 L over 24 hours in adults). Frequent urination is sometimes included by definition but is nonetheless usually an accompanying symptom. Increased production and passage of urine may also be termed dieresis

Polyuria often appears in conjunction with polydipsia (increased thirst), though it is possible to have one without the other, and the latter may be a cause or an effect.

Polyuria is physiologically normal in some circumstances, such as cold diuresis, altitude diuresis, and after drinking large amounts of fluids.

Causes

The most common cause of polyuria in both adults and children is uncontrolled diabetes mellitus, causing an osmotic diuresis. In the absence of diabetes mellitus, the most common causes are primary

polydipsia (excessive fluid drinking), central diabetes insipidus and nephrogenic diabetes insipidus. Polyuria may also be due to e.g. diabetes insipidus, hypercalcemia) or various chemical substances

(diuretics, caffeine, alcohol). Diuresis is restrained by antidiuretics such as ADH, angiotensin II and aldosterone.

Cold diuresis is the occurrence of increased urine production on exposure to cold, which also partially explains immersion diuresis.

Substances that increase diuresis are called diuretics.

Substances that decrease diuresis allow more vasopressin or antidiuretic hormone (ADH) to be present in the kidney.

High-altitude diuresis occurs at altitudes above 10,000 ft and is a desirable indicator of adaptation to high altitudes.

Other causes
increase in fluid intake, especially water
diuretic drugs
Diuretic foods (foods and beverages containing caffeine, such as chocolate, coffee, tea, and soft drinks; hot spicy foods; juices high in acid; alcoholic beverages; protein shakes, etc.)
diabetes mellitus
diabetes insipidus
Hypovolemia
Chronic Renal Failure

CHAPTER THREE

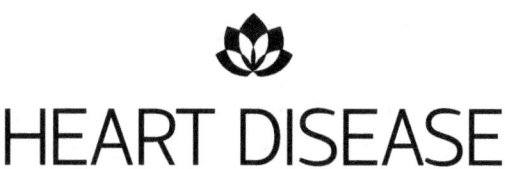

HEART DISEASE

Heart disease   -HISTORY TAKING AND SYMPTOMALOGY

Heart disease or cardiopathy is an umbrella term for a variety of diseases affecting the heart.
Types

Coronary heart disease

Coronary heart disease is the term used to refer to the failure of the coronary circulation to supply adequate circulation to cardiac muscle and its surrounding tissues. Coronary artery disease is a disease of the artery caused by the accumulation of atheromatous plaques within the walls of the arteries that supply the myocardium. Angina pectoris (chest pain) and myocardial infarction (heart attack) are symptoms of and conditions caused by coronary heart disease.

Cardiomyopathy

Cardiomyopathy Literally means "heart muscle disease" (Myo= muscle, pathy= disease) It is the deterioration of the function of the myocardium (i.e., the heart muscle) for any reason. People with cardiomyopathy are often at risk of arrhythmia and/or sudden cardiac death.

Extrinsic cardiomyopathies – cardiomyopathies where the primary pathology is outside the myocardium itself. Most cardiomyopathies are extrinsic because by far the most common cause of a cardiomyopathy are ischemia. The World Health Organization calls these specific cardiomyopathies Alcoholic cardiomyopathies

Coronary artery disease
Congenital heart disease
Nutritional diseases affecting the heart
Ischemic (or ischaemic) cardiomyopathy
Intrinsic cardiomyopathies – weakness in the muscle of the heart that is not due to an identifiable external cause.

Dilated cardiomyopathy (DCM) – most common form, and one of the leading indications for heart transplantation. In DCM the heart (especially the left ventricle) is enlarged and the pumping function is diminished.

Hypertrophic cardiomyopathy (HCM or HOCM) – genetic disorder caused by
various mutations in genes encoding sarcomere proteins. In HCM the heart muscle is thickened, which can obstruct blood flow and prevent the heart from functioning properly.

Arrhythmogenic right ventricular cardiomyopathy (ARVC) – arises from an electrical disturbance of the heart in which heart muscle is replaced by fibrous scar tissue. The right ventricle is generally most affected.

Restrictive cardiomyopathy (RCM) – least common cardiomyopathy. The walls of the ventricles are stiff, but may not be thickened, and resist the normal filling of the heart with blood.

Noncompaction Cardiomyopathy – the left ventricle wall has failed to properly grow from birth and such has a spongy appearance when viewed during an echocardiogram.

Cardiovascular disease

Cardiovascular disease is any of several specific diseases that affect the heart itself and/or the blood vessel system, especially the veins and arteries leading to and from the heart. Known or associated causes of cardiovascular disease include diabetes mellitus, hypertension, hyperhomocysteinemia and hypercholesterolemia.

Types of cardiovascular disease include:

Atherosclerosis

Ischaemic heart disease – another disease of the heart itself, characterized by the reduced blood supply to the organs.

Heart failure

Heart failure also called *congestive heart failure* (or *CHF*), and congestive cardiac failure (CCF), is a condition that can result from any structural or functional cardiac disorder that impairs the ability of the heart to fill with or pump a sufficient amount of blood throughout the body. Therefore, leading to the heart and body's failure.

Hypertensive heart disease

Hypertensive heart disease is heart disease caused by high blood pressure, especially localised high blood pressure. Conditions that can be caused by hypertensive heart disease include:
    Left ventricular hypertrophy
    Coronary heart disease
    Cardiac arrhythmias

Inflammatory heart disease

Inflammatory heart disease involves inflammation of the heart muscle and/or the tissue surrounding it.
    Endocarditis – inflammation of the inner layer of the heart, the endocardium. The most common structures involved are the heart valves.
    Inflammatory cardiomegaly
    Myocarditis – inflammation of the myocardium, the muscular part of the heart.

Valvular heart disease

Valvular heart disease is a disease process that affects one or more valves of the heart. There are four major heart valve which may be affected by valvular heart disease, including the tricuspid and aortic valves in the right side of the heart, as well as the mitral and aortic valves in the left side of the heart.

CHAPTER FOUR

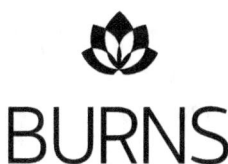

BURNS

BURNS-HISTORY TAKING AND SYMPTOMALOGY

A burn is a type of injury to flesh caused by heat, electricity, chemicals, light, radiation or friction. Most burns only affect the skin (or the epidermal tissue or dermis). Rarely, to the deeper tissues, such as muscle, bone, and blood vessels. Burns may be treated with first aid, in an out-of-hospital setting, or may require more specialized treatment such as those available at specialized burn centres.

Managing burns is important because they are common, painful and can result in disfiguring and disabling scarring, amputation of affected parts or death in severe cases. Complications such as shock, infection, multiple organ dysfunction syndrome, electrolyte imbalance and respiratory distress may occur. The treatment of burns may include the removal of dead tissue (debridement), applying dressings to the wound, administering large volumes of intravenous fluids, administering antibiotics and skin grafting.

Classification

Burns can be classified by mechanism of injury, depth, extent and associated injuries and comorbidities.

By depth

Currently, burns are described according to the depth of injury to the dermis and are loosely classified into first, second, third and fourth degrees. This system was devised by the French barber-surgeon Ambroise Pare and remains in use today.

It is often difficult to accurately determine the depth of a burn. This is especially so in the case of second-degree burns, which can continue to evolve over time. As such, a second- degree partial-thickness burn can progress to a third-degree burn over time even after initial treatment. Distinguishing between the superficial-thickness burn and the partial-thickness burn is important, as the former may heal spontaneously, whereas the latter often requires surgical excision and skin grafting.

By severity

In order to determine the need for referral to a specialized burn unit, the American Burn Association devised a classification system to aid in the decision-making process. Under this system, burns can be classified as major, moderate and minor. This is assessed based on a number of factors, including total body surface area (TBSA) burnt, the involvement of specific anatomical zones, age of the person and associated injuries.

Major

Major burns are defined as:
- Age 10-50yrs: partial thickness burns >25% of total body surface area
- Age <10 or >50: partial-thickness burns >20% of total body surface area
- Full-thickness burns >10%

Burns involving the hands, face, feet or perineum
Burns that cross major joints
Circumferential burns to any extremity
Any burn associated with inhalational injury
Electrical burns
Burns associated with fractures or other trauma
Burns in infants and the elderly
Burns in persons at high-risk of developing complications
These burns typically require referral to a specialized burn treatment center.

Moderate

Moderate burns are defined as:
Age 10-50yrs: partial thickness burns involving 15-25% of total body surface area
Age <10 or >50: partial thickness burns involving 10-20% of total body surface area
Full thickness burns involving 2-10% of total body surface area Persons suffering these burns often need to be hospitalized for burn care.

Minor

Minor burns are:
Age 10-50yrs: partial thickness burns <15% of total body surface area
Age <10 or >50: partial thickness burns involving <10% of total body surface area
Full thickness burns <2% of total body surface area, without associated injuries These burns usually do not require hospitalization.
By surface area
Burns can also be assessed in terms of total body surface area (TBSA), which is the percentage affected by partial-thickness or full-thickness burns. First degree (erythema only, no blisters) burns are not included in this estimation. The rule of nines is used as a quick and useful way to estimate the affected TBSA. More accurate estimation can be made using Lund & Browder charts which take into account the different proportions of body parts in adults and children. The size of a person's handprint (palm and fingers) is approximately 1% of their TBSA. The actual mean surface area is 0.8% so using 1% will slightly overestimate the size. Burns of 10% in children or 15% in adults (or greater) are potentially life-threatening injuries (because of the risk of hypovolemic shock) and should have formal fluid resuscitation and monitoring in a burn's unit.

Cause

Burns are caused by a wide variety of substances and external sources such as exposure to chemicals, friction, electricity, radiation, and heat.

Chemical

Most chemicals that cause chemical burns are strong acids or bases. Chemical burns can be caused by caustic chemical compounds such as sodium hydroxide or silver nitrate, and acids such as sulfuric acid Hydrofluoric acid can cause damage down to the bone and its burns are sometimes not immediately evident.

Electrical

Electrical burns are caused by either an electric shock or an uncontrolled short circuit. Lightning is also a rare cause of electrical burns.

Some electrocutions produce no external burns at all, as very little current is required to cause fibrillation of the heart muscle. Therefore, even when the injury does not involve any visible tissue damage, electrical shock survivors may experience significant internal injury.

Radiation

Radiation burns are caused by protracted exposure to UV light (as from the sun), tanning booths, radiation therapy (in people undergoing cancer therapy), sunlamps, radioactive fallout, and X-rays. By far the most common burn associated with radiation is sun exposure, specifically two wavelengths of light UVA, and UVB, the latter being more dangerous.

Tanning booths also emit these wavelengths and may cause similar damage to the skin such as irritation, redness, swelling, and inflammation. More severe cases of sunburn result in what is known as sun poisoning or "heatstroke". Microwave burns are caused by the thermal effects of microwave radiation.

Scalding

Scalding is derived from the Latin word *calidus*, meaning hot) is caused by hot liquids (water or oil) or gases (steam), most commonly occurring from exposure to high-temperature tap water in baths or showers or spilt hot drinks. A so-called *immersion scald* is created when an extremity is held under the surface of hot water and is a common form of burn seen in child abuse. A *blister* is a "bubble" in the skin filled with serous fluid as part of the body's reaction to the heat and the subsequent inflammatory reaction. The blister "roof" is dead and the blister fluid contains toxic inflammatory mediators. Scald burns are more common in children, especially "spill scalds" from hot drinks and bath water scalds.

Pathophysiology

Following a major burn injury, heart rate and peripheral vascular resistance increase. This is due to the release of catecholamines from injured tissues, and the relative hypovolemia that occurs from fluid volume shifts. Initially, cardiac output decreases. At approximately 24 hours after burn injuries, the cardiac output returns to normal if adequate fluid resuscitation has been given. Following this, cardiac output increases to meet the hypermetabolic needs of the body.

Management

The resuscitation phase begins with the reassessment of the injured person's airway, breathing and circulatory state. Appropriate interventions should be initiated to stabilize these. This may involve aggressive fluid resuscitation and, if inhalation injury is suspected, intubation. Once the injured person is stabilized, attention is turned to the care of the burn wound itself. Until then, it is advisable to cover the burn wound with a clean and dry sheet or dressing.

Early cooling reduces burn depth and pain, but care must be taken as uncontrolled cooling can result in hypothermia.

Intravenous fluids

Children with >10% total body surface area burns, and adults with >15% total body surface area burns need formal fluid resuscitation and monitoring (blood pressure, pulse rate, temperature and urine output). Once the burning process has been stopped, the injured person should be volume resuscitated according to the Parkland formula. This formula calculates the amount of Ringer's lactate required to be administered over the first 24hrs post-burn.

Parkland formula: 4mls x percentage total body surface area sustaining non-superficial burns x person's weight in kgs.

Half of this total volume should be administered over the first 8hrs, with the remainder given over the following 16hrs. It is important to note that this time frame is calculated from the time at which the burn is sustained, and not the time at which fluid resuscitation is begun.

Children also require the addition of maintenance fluid volume. Such injuries can disturb a person's osmotic balance. Inhalation injuries in conjunction with thermal burns initially require up to 40–50% more fluid.

The formula is a guide only and infusions must be tailored to the urine output and central venous pressure. Inadequate fluid resuscitation may cause renal failure and death but over- resuscitation also causes morbidity.

Wound care

Debridement cleaning and then dressings are important aspects of wound care. The wound should then be regularly re-evaluated until it is healed. In the management of first and second degree burns little quality evidence exists to determine which type of dressing should be used.

Antibiotics

Intravenous antibiotics may improve survival in those with large severe burns however due to the poor quality of the evidence routine use is not currently recommended.

Analgesics

A number of different options are used for pain management. These include simple analgesics (such as ibuprofen and acetaminophen) and narcotics. A local anesthetic may help in managing pain of minor first-degree and second-degree burns.

Surgery

Wounds requiring surgical closure with skin grafts or flaps should be dealt with as early as possible. Circumferential burns of digits, limbs or the chest may need urgent surgical release of the burnt skin (escharotomy) to prevent problems with distal circulation or ventilation.

Alternative treatments

Hyperbaric oxygenation has not been shown to be a useful adjunct to traditional treatments. Honey has been used since ancient times to aid wound healing and may be beneficial in first- and second-degree burns, but may cause infection.

Complications

Infection is a major complication of burns. Infection is linked to impaired resistance from disruption of the skin's mechanical integrity and generalized immune suppression. The skin barrier is replaced by eschar. This moist, protein rich avascular environment encourages microbial growth. Migration of immune cells is hampered, and there is a release of intermediaries that impede the immune response. Eschar also restricts distribution of systemically administered antibiotics because of its avascularity.

Risk factors of burn wound infection include:
Burn > 30% TBS
Full-thickness burn
Extremes in age (very young, very old)
Preexisting disease e.g. diabetes
Virulence and antibiotic resistance of colonizing organism
Failed skin graft
Improper initial burn wound care

Prolonged open burn wound

Burn wounds are prone to tetanus. A tetanus booster shot is required if an individual has not been immunized within the last 5 years.

Prognosis

The outcome of any injury or disease depends on three things: the nature of the injury, the nature of the injured or ill person and the treatment available. In terms of injury factors in burns, the prognosis depends primarily on total body surface area percentage and the age of the person. The presence of smoke inhalation injury, other significant injuries such as long bone fractures and serious co-morbidities (heart disease, diabetes, psychiatric illness, suicidal intent etc.) will also adversely influence prognosis. Advances in resuscitation, surgical management, control of infection, control of the hyper-metabolic response and rehabilitation have resulted in dramatic improvements in burn mortality and morbidity in the last 60 years.

Epidemiology

Demographically, In India about 700,000 people a year are admitted to hospital, though very few are looked after in specialist burn units.

About 90% of burns occur in the developing world and 70% of these are in children. Survival of injuries greater than 40% total body surface area is rare in the developing world.

CHAPTER FIVE

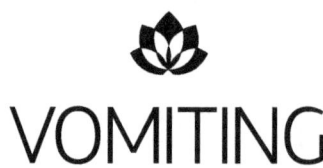

VOMITING

Vomiting -HISTORY TAKING AND SYMPTOMALOGY

Vomiting (also known medically as emesis and informally as throwing up and by a number of other terms) is the forceful expulsion of the contents of one's stomach through the mouth and sometimes the nose. Vomiting can occur due to a wide variety of conditions; it may present as a specific response to ailments like gastritis or poisoning, or as a non-specific sequela of disorders

The feeling that one is about to vomit is called nausea, which usually precedes, but does not always lead to vomiting. Antiemetics are sometimes necessary to suppress nausea and vomiting. In severe cases, where dehydration develops, intravenous fluid may be required.

Vomiting is different from regurgitation, although the two terms are often used interchangeably. Regurgitation is the return of undigested food back up the esophagus to the mouth, without the force and displeasure associated with vomiting. The causes of vomiting and regurgitation are generally different.

Complications

Aspiration of vomit

Vomiting can be dangerous if the gastric content gets into the respiratory tract. Under normal circumstances the gag reflex and this from occurring, however these protective reflexes are compromised in persons under the influences of certain substances such as alcohol or anesthesia. The individual may choke and asphyxiate or suffer an aspiration pneumonia.

Dehydration and electrolyte imbalance

Prolonged and excessive vomiting depletes the body of water (dehydration), and may alter the electrolyte status. Gastric vomiting leads to the loss of acid (protons) and chlorine directly. Combined with the resulting alkaline tide, this lead to hypochloremia metabolic alkalosis (low chloride levels together with high HCO_3 and CO_2 and increased blood pH) and often hypokalemia (potassium depletion). The hypokalemia is an indirect result of the kidney compensating for the loss of acid. With the loss of intake of food the individual may eventually become cachectic. A less frequent occurrence results from a vomiting of intestinal contents, including bile acids and HCO_3-, which can lead to metabolic acidosis.

Mallory-Weiss tear

Repeated or profuse vomiting may cause erosions to the oesophagus or small tears in the oesophagal mucosa (Mallory-Weiss tear).

This may become apparent if fresh red blood is mixed with vomit after several episodes.

Dentistry

Recurrent vomiting, such as observed in bulimia nervosa, may lead to the destruction of the tooth enamel due to the acidity of the Vomit, Digestive enzymes can also have a negative effect on oral health, by degrading the tissue of the gums.

Pathophysiology

Receptors on the floor of the fourth ventricle of the brain represent a chemoreceptor trigger zone, known as the area postrema, stimulation of which can lead to vomiting. The area postrema is a circumventricular organ and as such lies outside the blood-brain barrier; it can, therefore, be stimulated by blood-borne drugs that can stimulate vomiting or inhibit it.

There are various sources of input to the vomiting center:

The chemoreceptor trigger zone at the base of the fourth ventricle has numerous dopamine D2receptors, serotonin 5- HT3 receptors, opioid receptors, acetylcholine receptors, and receptors for substance P. Stimulation of different receptors are involved in different pathways leading to emesis, in the final common pathway substance P appears involved.

The vestibular system, which sends information to the brain via cranial nerve VIII (vestibulocochlear nerve), plays a major role in motion sickness and is rich in muscarinic receptors and histamine H1 receptors.

The Cranial nerve X (vagus nerve) is activated when the pharynx is irritated, leading to a gag reflex.

The Vagal and enteric nervous system inputs transmit information regarding the state of the gastrointestinal system.

Irritation of the GI mucosa by chemotherapy, radiation, distention, or acute infectious gastroenteritis activates the 5- HT3 receptors of these inputs.

The CNS mediates vomiting that arises from psychiatric disorders and stress from higher brain centers.

The vomiting act encompasses three types of outputs initiated by the chemoreceptor trigger zone: Motor, parasympathetic nervous system (PNS), and sympathetic nervous system (SNS). They are as follows:

Increased salivation to protect tooth enamel from stomach acids. (Excessive vomiting leads to dental erosion). This is part of the PNS output.

The body takes a deep breath to avoid aspirating vomit.

Retro peristalsis, starts from the middle of the small intestine and sweeps up digestive tract contents into the stomach, through the relaxed pyloric sphincter.

Intrathoracic pressure lowers (by inspiration against a closed glottis), coupled with an increase in abdominal pressure as the abdominal muscles contract, propels stomach contents into the esophagus as the lower esophageal sphincter relaxes. The stomach itself does not contract in the process of vomiting except for at the angular notch, nor is there any retro peristalsis in the esophagus.

Vomiting is ordinarily preceded by retching.

Vomiting also initiates an SNS response causing both sweating and increased heart rate.

The neurotransmitters that regulate vomiting are poorly understood, but inhibitors of dopamine, histamine, and serotonin are all used to suppress vomiting, suggesting that these play a role in the initiation or maintenance of a vomiting cycle. Vasopressin and neurokinin may also participate.

Phases

The vomiting act has two phases. In the retching phase, the abdominal muscles undergo a few rounds of coordinated contractions together with the diaphragm and the muscles used in respiratory inspiration. For this reason, an individual may confuse this phase with an episode of violent hiccups. In this retching phase nothing has yet been expelled. In the next phase, also termed the expulsive phase, intense pressure is formed in the stomach brought about by enormous shifts in both the diaphragm and the abdomen. These shifts are, in essence, vigorous contractions of these muscles that last for extended periods of time - much longer than a normal period of muscular contraction. The pressure is then suddenly released when the upper esophageal sphincter relaxes resulting in the expulsion of gastric contents. For people not in the habit of exercising the abdominal muscles, they may be painful for the next few days. The relief of pressure and the release of endorphins into the bloodstream after the expulsion causes the vomited to feel better.

Contents

Gastric secretions and likewise vomit are highly acidic. Recent food intake appears in the gastric vomit. Irrespective of the content, vomit tends to be malodorous.

The content of the *vomitus* (vomit) may be of medical interest. Fresh blood in the vomit is termed hematemesis ("blood vomiting").

Altered blood bears resemblance to coffee grounds (as the iron in the blood is oxidized) and, when this matter is identified, the term "coffee ground vomiting" is used. Bile can enter the vomit during subsequent heaves due to duodenal contraction if the vomiting is severe. Fecal vomiting is often a consequence of intestinal obstruction or a gastrocolic fistula and is treated as a warning sign of this potentially serious problem such vomiting is sometimes called "miserere."

If the vomiting reflex continues for an extended period with no appreciable vomitus, the condition is known as *non-productive emesis* or *dry heaves*, which can be painful and debilitating.

Color of vomit-Bright red in the vomit suggests bleeding from the esophagus

Dark red vomit with liver-like clots suggests profuse bleeding in the stomach, such as from a perforated ulcer Coffee ground-like vomit suggests less severe bleeding in the stomach, because the gastric acid has had time to change the composition of the blood Yellow vomit suggests bile. This indicates that the pyloric valve is open and bile is flowing into the stomach from the duodenum. (This is more common in older people.)

Differential diagnosis

Vomiting may be due to a large number of causes, and protracted vomiting has a long differential diagnosis.
- Digestive tract
- Causes in the digestive tract
- Gastritis (inflammation of the gastric wall, usually by viruses)
- Gastroenteritis
- Food allergies (often in conjunction with hives or swelling)
- Cholecystitis, pancreatitis, appendicitis, hepatitis
- Food poisoning
- In children, it can be caused by an allergic reaction to cow's milk proteins (Milk allergy or lactose intolerance)
- Sensory system and brain
- Causes in the sensory system
- Movement: motion sickness (which is caused by overstimulation of the labyrinthine canals of the ear)
- Causes in the brain
- concussion
- Cerebral hemorrhage
- Migraine
- Brain tumors, which can cause the chemoreceptors to malfunction
- Benign intracranial hypertension and hydrocephalus
- Metabolic disturbances (these may irritate both the stomach and the parts of the brain that coordinate vomiting)
- Hypercalcemia (high calcium levels)
- Uremia (urea accumulation, usually due to renal failure)
- Hyperemesis, Morning sickness
- Drug reaction (vomiting may occur as an acute somatic response to)
- alcohol (being sick while being drunk or being sick the next morning, suffering from the after-effects, i.e., the hangover).

opioids
selective serotonin reuptake inhibitors
many chemotherapies drug
some entheogens (such as peyote or ayahuasca)
Illness (sometimes colloquially known as "stomach flu"—a broad name that refers to gastric inflammation caused by a range of viruses and bacteria.)
Norovirus (Formerly Norwalk virus or Norwalk agent)
Swine Flu

Emetics

An *emetic* is a substance that induces vomiting when administered orally or by injection. An emetic is used medically where a substance has been ingested and must be expelled from the body immediately (for this reason, many toxic and easily digestible products such as rat poison contain an emetic). Inducing vomiting can remove the substance before it is absorbed into the body. Ipecac abuse can cause detrimental health effects.

Salt water and mustard water have been used since ancient times as emetics. Care must be taken with salt, as excessive intake can potentially be harmful. Copper sulfate was also used in the past as an emetic. It is now considered too toxic for this use

Miscellanea
Self-induced
Eating disorders (anorexia nervosa or bulimia nervosa)
To eliminate an ingested poison (some poisons should not be vomited as they may be more toxic when inhaled or aspirated; it is better to ask for help before inducing vomiting)
Some people who engage in binge drinking induce vomiting to make room in their stomachs for more alcohol consumption.
People suffering from nausea may induce vomiting in hopes of feeling better.
After surgery (postoperative nausea and vomiting)
Disagreeable sights, smells or thoughts (such as decayed matter, others' vomit, thinking of vomiting), etc.
Extreme pain, such as intense headache or myocardial infarction (heart attack)
Violent emotions
Cyclic vomiting syndrome (a poorly-understood condition with attacks of vomiting)
Nervousness
Anxiety
Overexertion (doing too much strenuous exercise can lead to vomiting shortly afterwards).

Treatment

An antiemetic is a drug that is effective against vomiting and nausea. Antiemetics are typically used to treat motion sickness and the side-effects of medications such as opioids and chemotherapy.

Antiemetics act by inhibiting the receptor sites associated with emesis. Hence, anticholinergics, antihistamines, dopamine antagonists, serotonin antagonists, and cannabinoids are used as anti-emetics.

CHAPTER SIX

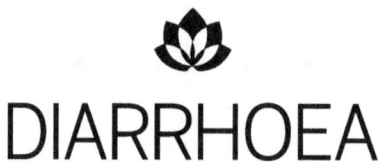

DIARRHOEA

Diarrhoea-HISTORY TAKING AND SYMPTOMALOGY
is the condition of having three or more loose or liquid bowel movements per day. It is a common cause of death in developing countries and the second most common cause of infant deaths worldwide. The loss of fluids through diarrhea can cause dehydration and electrolyte imbalances.

Definition

Diarrhea is defined by the World Health Organization as having 3 or more loose or liquid stools per day, or as having more stools than is normal for that person.

Secretory

Secretory diarrhea means that there is an increase in the active secretion, or there is an inhibition of absorption. There is little to no structural damage. The most common cause of this type of diarrhea is a cholera toxin that stimulates the secretion of anions, especially chloride ions. Therefore, to maintain a charge balance in the lumen, sodium is carried with it, along with water. In this type of diarrhea intestinal fluid secretion is isotonic with plasma even during fasting. It continues even when there is no oral food intake.
Osmotic
Osmotic diarrhea occurs when too much water is drawn into the bowels. This can be the result of maldigestion (e.g., pancreatic disease or celiac disease), in which the nutrients are left in the lumen to pull in water. Osmotic diarrhea can also be caused by osmotic laxatives (which work to alleviate constipation by drawing water into the bowels). In healthy individuals, too much magnesium or vitamin C or undigested lactose can produce osmotic diarrhea and distention of the bowel. A person who has lactose intolerance can have difficulty absorbing lactose after an extraordinarily high intake of dairy products. In persons who have fructose malabsorption, excess fructose intake can also cause diarrhea. High-fructose foods that also have a high glucose content are more absorbable and less likely to cause diarrhea. Sugar alcohols such as sorbitol (often found in sugar-free foods) are difficult for the body to absorb and, in large amounts, may lead to osmotic diarrhea. Osmotic diarrhea stops when offending agent (e.g. milk, sorbitol) is stopped.

Exudative

Exudative diarrhea occurs with the presence of blood and pus in the stool. This occurs with inflammatory bowel diseases, such as Crohn's disease or ulcerative colitis, and other severe infections such as *E. coli* or other forms of food poisoning.
Motility-related
Motility-related diarrhea is caused by the rapid movement of food through the intestines (hypermotility). If the food moves too quickly through the gastrointestinal tract, there is not enough time for sufficient nutrients and water to be absorbed. This can be due to a vagotomy or diabetic neuropathy, or a complication of

menstruation. Hyperthyroidism can produce hypermotility and lead to pseudo-diarrhea and occasionally real diarrhea. Diarrhea can be treated with antimotility agents (such as loperamide). Hypermotility can be observed in people who have had portions of their bowel removed, allowing less total time for absorption of nutrients.

Inflammatory

Inflammatory diarrhea occurs when there is damage to the mucosal lining or brush border, which leads to a passive loss of protein-rich fluids, and a decreased ability to absorb these lost fluids. Features of all three of the other types of diarrhea can be found in this type of diarrhea. It can be caused by bacterial infections, viral infections, parasitic infections, or autoimmune problems such as inflammatory bowel diseases. It can also be caused by tuberculosis, colon cancer, and enteritis

Dysentery

Generally, if there is blood visible in the stools, it is not diarrhea, but dysentery. The blood is trace of an invasion of bowel tissue. Dysentery is a symptom of, among others, *Shigella, Entamoeba histolytica*, and *Salmonella*.

Differential diagnosis

Diarrhea is most commonly due to viral gastroenteritis with rotavirus, which accounts for 40% of cases in children under five.

Chronic diarrhea can be the part of the presentations of a number of chronic medical conditions affecting the intestine. Common causes include ulcerative colitis, Crohn's disease, microscopic colitis, celiac disease, irritable bowel syndrome and bile acid malabsorption.

Infections

There are many causes of infectious diarrhea, which include viruses, bacteria and parasites. Norovirus is the most common cause of viral diarrhea in adults, but rotavirus is the most common cause in children under five years old.

The bacterium Campylobacter is a common cause of bacterial diarrhea, but infections by Salmonellae, Shigella and some strains of *Escherichia coli* (E. coli) are frequent.

In the elderly, particularly those who have been treated with antibiotics for unrelated infections, a toxin produced by *Clostridium difficile* often causes severe diarrhea.

Parasites do not often cause diarrhea except for the protozoan *Giardia*, which can cause chronic infections if these are not diagnosed and treated with drugs such as metronidazole, and *Entamoeba histolytica*.

Other infectious agents such as parasites and bacterial toxins also occur. In sanitary living conditions where there is ample food and a supply of clean water, an otherwise healthy person usually recovers from viral infections in a few days. However, for ill or malnourished individuals, diarrhea can lead to severe dehydration and can become life-threatening.

Malabsorption

Malabsorption is the inability to absorb food fully, mostly from disorders in the small bowel, but also due to maldigestion from diseases of the pancreas.

Causes include:

enzyme deficiencies or mucosal abnormality, as in food allergy and food intolerance, (e.g. celiac disease (gluten intolerance), lactose intolerance (intolerance to milk sugar, common in non-Europeans), fructose malabsorption) pernicious anemia (impaired bowel function due to the inability to absorb vitamin B_{12}), loss of pancreatic secretions (may be due to cystic fibrosis or pancreatitis), structural defects, like short bowel syndrome (surgically removed bowel) and radiation fibrosis (usually following cancer treatment and other drugs, including agents used in chemotherapy), certain drugs (like orlistat, which inhibits the absorption of fat).

Inflammatory bowel disease

The two overlapping types here are of unknown origin:

Ulcerative colitis is marked by chronic bloody diarrhea and inflammation mostly affects the distal colon near the rectum.

Crohn's disease typically affects fairly well-demarcated segments of bowel in the colon and often affects the end of the small bowel.

Irritable bowel syndrome

Another possible cause of diarrhea is irritable bowel syndrome (IBS) which usually presents with abdominal discomfort relieved by defecation and unusual stool (diarrhea or constipation) for at least 3 days a week over the previous 3 months. Symptoms of diarrhea-predominant IBS can be managed through a combination of dietary changes, soluble fiber supplements, and/or medications such as loperamide or codeine.

Other causes

Diarrhea can be caused by chronic ethanol ingestion.

Ischemic bowel disease. This usually affects older people and can be due to blocked arteries.

Microscopic colitis, a type of inflammatory bowel disease where changes are only seen on histological examination of colonic biopsies.

Bile salt malabsorption (primary bile acid diarrhea) where excessive bile acids in the colon produce a secretory diarrhea.

Hormone-secreting tumors: some hormones (e.g., serotonin) can cause diarrhea if excreted in excess (usually from a tumor).

Chronic mild diarrhea in infants and toddlers may occur with no obvious cause and with no other ill effects; this condition is called toddler's diarrhea.

Pathophysiology

Diagnostic approach

The following types of diarrhea may indicate further investigation is needed:

In infants

Moderate or severe diarrhea in young children

Associated with blood

Continues for more than two days

Associated non-cramping abdominal pain, fever, weight loss, etc.

In travelers

In food handlers, because of the potential to infect others;

In institutions such as hospitals, child care centers, or geriatric and convalescent homes.

A severity score is used to aid diagnosis in children.

Prevention

A rotavirus vaccine has the potential to decrease rates of diarrhea. There are currently two licensed vaccines against rotavirus. New vaccines against rotavirus, *Shigella*, ETEC, and cholera are under development, as well as other causes of infectious diarrhea.

A Cochrane Review of studies found that in institutions and in communities, interventions that promote hand washing lead to significant reductions in the incidence of diarrhea.

Management

In many cases of diarrhea, replacing lost fluid and salts is the only treatment needed. This is usually by mouth – oral rehydration therapy – or, in severe cases, intravenously

Diet restrictions such as the BRAT diet are no longer recommended. Research does not support the limiting of milk to children as doing so has no effect on duration of diarrhea.

Medications such as loperamide (Imodium), bismuth subsalicylate may be beneficial, however they may be contraindicated in certain situations.

Medications

Antibiotics

While antibiotics are beneficial in certain type of acute diarrhea they are usually not used except in specific situations. There are concerns that antibiotics may increase the risk of hemolytic uremic syndrome in people infected with Escherichia coil O157:H7. In resource poor countries treatment with antibiotics may be beneficial. However, some bacteria are developing antibiotic resistance, particularly *Shigella*.

Bismuth compounds

While bismuth compounds (Pepto-Bismol) decreased the number of bowel movements in those with travelers' diarrhea it does not decrease the length of illness. These agents should only be used if bloody diarrhea is not present.

Anti-motility agents

Anti-motility agents like loperamide are effective at reducing the duration of diarrhea.

Codeine phosphate

Codeine phosphate is used in the treatment of diarrhea to slow down Peristalsis and the passage of fecal material through the bowels - this means that more time is given for water to reabsorb back into the body, which gives a firmer stool, and also means that feces are passed less frequently.

Zinc

A Cochrane systematic review found that zinc supplementation benefits children suffering from diarrhea in developing countries, but only in infants over six months old. This supports the World Health Organization guidelines for zinc, but not in the very young.

Bile acid sequestrants

Bile acid sequestrants such as cholestyramine, colestipol and Colesville can be effective in chronic diarrhea due to bile acid malabsorption.

CHAPTER SEVEN

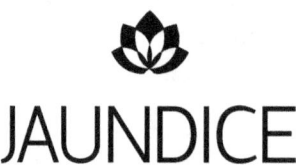

JAUNDICE

Jaundice is a yellowish pigmentation of the skin, the conjunctival membranes over the sclerae (whites of the eyes), and their mucous membranes caused by hyperbilirubinemia (increased levels of bilirubin in the blood). This hyperbilirubinemia subsequently causes increased levels of bilirubin in the extracellular fluid. Typically, the concentration of bilirubin in plasma must exceed 1.5 mg/dL (>26μmol/L), three times the usual value of approximately 0.5 mg/dL for the colouration to be easily visible. Jaundice comes from the French word *jaune*, meaning yellow.

Jaundice is often seen in liver diseases such as hepatitis or liver cancer. It may also indicate obstruction of the biliary tract, for example by gallstones or pancreatic cancer, or less commonly be congenital in origin.

Icterus

The conjunctiva of the eye is one of the first tissues to change color as bilirubin levels rise in jaundice. This is sometimes referred to as *scleral icterus*. However, the sclera themselves are not "icteric" (stained with bile pigment) but rather the conjunctival membranes that overlie them. The yellowing of the "white of the eye" is thus more properly termed *conjunctival icterus*. The term "icterus" itself is sometimes incorrectly used to refer to jaundice that is noted in the sclera of the eyes, however its more common and more correct meaning is entirely synonymous with jaundice.

Differential diagnosis

When a pathological process interferes with the normal functioning of the metabolism and excretion of bilirubin just described, jaundice may be the result. Jaundice is classified into three categories, depending on which part of the physiological mechanism the pathology affects. The three categories are:

Category

The pathology is located after the conjugation of bilirubin in the liver.

Pre-hepatic

Pre-hepatic jaundice is caused by anything which causes an increased rate of hemolysis (breakdown of red blood cells). In tropical countries, malaria can cause jaundice in this manner. Certain genetic diseases, such as sickle cell anemia, spherocytosis, thalassemia and glucose 6-phosphate dehydrogenase deficiency can lead to increased red cell lysis and therefore hemolytic jaundice. Commonly, diseases of the kidney, such as hemolytic uremic syndrome, can also lead to coloration.

Defects in bilirubin metabolism also present as jaundice, as in Gilbert's syndrome (a genetic disorder of bilirubin metabolism which can result in mild jaundice, which is found in about 5% of the population) and Cigler-Najjar syndrome.

In jaundice secondary to hemolysis, the increased production of bilirubin, leads to the increased production of urine-urobilinogen. Bilirubin is not usually found in the urine because unconjugated bilirubin is not water-soluble, so, the combination of increased urine-urobilinogen with no bilirubin (since, unconjugated) in urine is suggestive of hemolytic jaundice.

Laboratory findings include:

Urine: no bilirubin present, azobilirubin > 2 units (i.e., hemolytic anaemia causes increased heme metabolism; exception: infants where gut flora has not developed).

Serum: increased unconjugated bilirubin.

Kernicterus is associated with increased unconjugated bilirubin.

Hepatocellular

Hepatocellular (hepatic) jaundice can be caused by acute hepatitis, hepatotoxicity, and alcoholic liver disease. Cell necrosis reduces the liver's ability to metabolize and excrete bilirubin leading to a buildup of unconjugated bilirubin in the blood. Other causes include primary biliary cirrhosis leading to an increase in plasma conjugated bilirubin.

Jaundice seen in the newborn, known as neonatal jaundice, is common, occurring in almost every newborn as hepatic machinery for the conjugation and excretion of bilirubin does not fully mature until approximately two weeks of age. Rat fever (leptospirosis) can also cause hepatic jaundice. In hepatic jaundice, there is invariably cholestasis.

Laboratory findings depend on the cause of jaundice.

Urine: Conjugated bilirubin present, azobilirubin > 2 units but variable (except in children). Kernicterus is a condition not associated with increased conjugated bilirubin.

Post-hepatic

Post-hepatic jaundice, also called obstructive jaundice, is caused by an interruption to the drainage of bile in the biliary system. The most common causes are gallstones in the common bile duct, and pancreatic cancer in the head of the pancreas. Also, a group of parasites known as "liver flukes" can live in the common bile duct, causing obstructive jaundice.

In complete obstruction of the bile duct, no urobilinogen is found in the urine, since bilirubin has no access to the intestine and it's in the intestine that bilirubin gets converted to urobilinogen to be later released into the general circulation. In this case, the presence of bilirubin(conjugated) in the urine without urine-urobilinogen suggests obstructive jaundice, either intra-hepatic or post-hepatic.

The presence of pale stools and dark urine suggests an obstructive or post-hepatic cause as normal feces get their color from bile pigments. However, although pale stools and dark urine are a feature of biliary obstruction, they can occur in many intra-hepatic illnesses and are therefore not a reliable clinical feature to distinguish obstruction from hepatic causes of jaundice.

Patients also can present with elevated serum cholesterol, and often complain of severe itching or "pruritus" because of the deposition of bile salts.

No single test can differentiate between various classifications of jaundice. A combination of liver function tests is essential to arrive at a diagnosis.

Neonatal jaundice

Neonatal jaundice is usually harmless: this condition is often seen in infants around the second day after birth, lasting until day 8 in normal births, or to around day 14 in premature births. Serum bilirubin normally drops to a low level without any intervention required: the jaundice is presumably a consequence of metabolic and physiological adjustments after birth. In extreme cases, a brain-damaging condition known as kernicterus can occur, leading to significant lifelong disability; there are concerns that this condition has been rising in recent years due to inadequate detection and treatment of neonatal hyperbilirubinemia.

A Bili light is often the tool used for early treatment, which often consists of exposing the baby to intensive phototherapy. Bilirubin count is lowered through bowel movements and urination so regular and proper feedings are especially important.

Pathophysiology

In order to understand how jaundice results, the pathological processes that cause jaundice to take their effect must be understood. Jaundice itself is not a disease, but rather a sign of one of many possible underlying pathological processes that occur at some point along the normal physiological pathway of the metabolism of bilirubin.

When red blood cells have completed their life span of approximately 120 days, or when they are damaged, their membranes become fragile and prone to rupture. As each red blood cell traverses through the reticuloendothelial system, its cell membrane ruptures when its membrane is fragile enough to allow this. Cellular contents, including hemoglobin, are subsequently released into the blood. The hemoglobin is phagocytosed by macrophages, and split into its heme and globin portions. The globin portion, a protein, is degraded into amino acids and plays no role in jaundice. Two reactions then take place with the heme molecule. The first oxidation reaction is catalyzed by the microsomal enzyme heme oxygenase and results in biliverdin (green colour pigment), iron and carbon monoxide. The next step is the reduction of biliverdin to a yellow colour tetrapyrrole pigment called bilirubin by cytosolic enzyme biliverdin reductase. This bilirubin is "unconjugated," "free" or "indirect" bilirubin. Approximately 4 mg per kg of bilirubin is produced each day. The majority of this bilirubin comes from the breakdown of heme from expired red blood cells in the process just described. However, approximately 20 per cent comes from other heme sources, including ineffective erythropoiesis, and the breakdown of other heme-containing proteins, such as muscle myoglobin and cytochromes.

Hepatic events

The unconjugated bilirubin then travels to the liver through the bloodstream. Because this bilirubin is not soluble, however, it is transported through the blood bound to serum albumin. Once it arrives at the liver, it is conjugated with glucuronic acid (to form bilirubin diglucuronide, or just "conjugated bilirubin") to become more water soluble. The reaction is catalyzed by the enzyme UDP-glucuronic transferase.

This conjugated bilirubin is excreted from the liver into the biliary and cystic ducts as part of bile. Intestinal bacteria convert the bilirubin into urobilinogen. From here the urobilinogen can take two pathways. It can either be further converted into stercobilin, which is then oxidized to stercobilin and passed out in the feces, or it can be reabsorbed by the intestinal cells, transported in the blood to the kidneys, and passed out in the urine as the oxidized product urobilin. Stercobilin and urobilin are the products responsible for the colouration of faeces and urine, respectively.

Most patients presenting with jaundice will have various predictable patterns of liver panel abnormalities, though significant variation does exist. The typical liver panel will include blood levels of enzymes found primarily from the liver, such as the aminotransferases (ALT, AST), and alkaline phosphatase (ALP); bilirubin (which causes jaundice); and protein levels, specifically, total protein and albumin. Other primary lab tests for liver function include GGT and prothrombin time (PT).

Some bone and heart disorders can lead to an increase in ALP and the aminotransferases, so the first step in differentiating these from liver problems is to compare the levels of GGT, which will only be elevated in liver-specific conditions. The second step is distinguishing from biliary (cholestatic) or liver (hepatic) causes of jaundice and altered lab results. The former typically indicates a surgical response, while the latter typically leans toward a medical response. ALP and GGT levels will typically rise with one pattern while AST and ALT rise in a separate pattern. If the ALP (10–45 IU/L) and GGT (18–85) levels rise proportionately about as high as the AST (12–38 IU/L) and ALT (10–45 IU/L) levels, this indicates a cholestatic problem. On the other hand, if the AST and ALT rise is significantly higher than the ALP and GGT rise, this indicates a hepatic problem. Finally, distinguishing between hepatic causes of jaundice, comparing levels of AST and ALT can prove useful.

AST levels will typically be higher than ALT. This remains the case in most hepatic disorders except for hepatitis (viral or hepatotoxic). Alcoholic liver damage may see fairly normal ALT levels, with AST 10x higher than ALT. On the other hand, if ALT is higher than AST, this is indicative of hepatitis. Levels of ALT and AST are not well correlated to the extent of liver damage, although rapid drops in these levels from very high levels can indicate severe necrosis. Low levels of albumin tend to indicate a chronic condition, while it is normal in hepatitis and cholestasis.

Complications

Complications of jaundice include sepsis especially cholangitis, biliary cirrhosis, pancreatitis, coagulopathy, renal and liver failure. Other complications are related to the underlying disease and the procedures employed in the diagnosis and management of individual diseases. Cholangitis especially the suppurative type (Charcot's triad or Raynaud's pentad) is usually secondary to choledocholithiasis. It may also complicate procedures like ERCP. Treatment should include correction of coagulopathy, fluid/electrolyte anomaly, antibiotics and biliary drainage with ERCP where available or trans-hepatic drainage or surgery.

Epistaxis

Epistaxis is derived from Greek word to bleed from the nose "to drip" [from the nostrils]) or a nosebleed is the relatively common occurrence of hemorrhage from the nose, usually noticed when the blood drains out through the nostrils. There are two types: anterior (the most common), and posterior (less common, more likely to require medical attention). Sometimes in more severe cases, the blood can come up the nasolacrimal duct and out from the eye. Fresh blood and clotted blood can also flow down into the stomach and cause nausea and vomiting.

Cause

The causes of nosebleeds can generally be divided into two categories, local and systemic factors, although it should be remembered that a significant number of nosebleeds occur with no obvious cause.

Local factors

Blunt trauma (usually a sharp blow to the face such as a punch, sometimes accompanying a nasal fracture) Foreign bodies (such as fingers during nose-picking)

Inflammatory reaction (*e.g.* acute respiratory tract infections, chronic sinusitis, allergic rhinitis or environmental irritants)

Other possible factors

Anatomical deformities (*e.g.* septal spurs or Hereditary hemorrhagic telangiectasia)

Insufflated drugs (particularly cocaine)

Intranasal tumors (*e.g.* Nasopharyngeal carcinoma or nasopharyngeal angiofibroma)

Low relative humidity of inhaled air (particularly during cold winter seasons)

Nasal cannula O_2 (tending to dry the olfactory mucosa)

Nasal sprays (particularly prolonged or improper use of nasal steroids)

Otic barotrauma (such as from descent in aircraft or ascent in scuba diving)

Surgery (*e.g.* septoplasty and Functional Endoscopic Sinus Surgery)

Leech infestation

Systemic factors

Most common factors

Allergies

Infectious diseases (*e.g.* common cold)

Hypertension

Other possible factors

Drugs —

Aspirin, Fexofenadine/Allegra/Telfast, warfarin, ibuprofen, clopidogrel, prasugrel, isotretinoin, desmopressin, ginseng and others

Alcohol (due to vasodilation)

Anemia

Connective tissue disease

Idiopathic thrombocytopenic purpura
Pregnancy (rare)
Vascular disorders
Vitamin C or Vitamin K deficiency
von Willebrand's disease

Pathophysiology

Nosebleeds are due to the rupture of a blood vessel within the richly perfused nasal mucosa. Rupture may be spontaneous or initiated by trauma. An increase in blood pressure (e.g. due to general hypertension) tends to increase the duration of spontaneous epistaxis. Anticoagulant medication and disorders of blood clotting can promote and prolong bleeding. Spontaneous epistaxis is more common in the elderly as the nasal mucosa (lining) becomes dry and thin and blood pressure tends to be higher.

Treatment

The flow of blood normally stops when the blood clots, which may be encouraged by direct pressure applied by pinching the soft fleshy part of the nose. This applies pressure to Little's area (Kiesselbach's area), the source of the majority of nose bleeds and promotes clotting. Pressure should be firm and be applied for at least five minutes and up to 20 minutes; tilting the head forward will help decrease the chance of nausea and airway obstruction. Swallowing excess blood can irritate the stomach and cause vomiting. Local application of an ice pack to the forehead or back of the neck or sucking an ice cube has seen widespread practice but has been shown to not have any statistically significant effects on nasal mucosal blood flow. There are conflicting opinions in the use of ice or nasal packing in the treatment of nose bleeds. Most suggest there is no detriment to using ice or nasal packing when initial efforts to pinch the nose fail, while others advise against it.

The local application of a vasoconstrictive agent has been shown to reduce the bleeding time in benign cases of epistaxis. The drugs oxymetazoline or phenylephrine are widely available in over-the-counter nasal sprays for the treatment of allergic rhinitis and may be used for this purpose.

If these simple measures do not work then medical intervention may be needed to stop bleeding, possibly by an otolaryngologist (ENT doctor). In the first instance, this can take the form of chemical cautery of any bleeding vessels or packing of the nose with ribbon gauze or an absorbent dressing (called anterior nasal packing).

Application of a topical antibiotic ointment to the nasal mucosa has been shown to be an effective treatment for recurrent epistaxis.

Recurrent nosebleeds may cause anaemia due to iron deficiency.

CHAPTER EIGHT

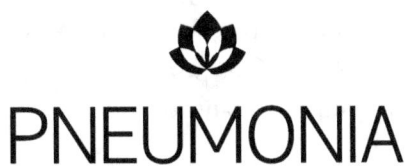

PNEUMONIA

Pneumonia is an inflammatory condition of the lung, especially of the alveoli (microscopic air sacs in the lungs) associated with fever, chest symptoms, and consolidation on a chest radiograph. While typically caused by an infection there are a number of noninfectious causes. infecting agents include bacteria, viruses, fungi, and parasites. Noninfectious causes include chemical burns, physical injury, drug reactions and vascular complications

Typical symptoms include cough, chest pain, fever, and difficulty breathing Diagnostic tools include x-rays and examination of the sputum. Vaccines to prevent certain types of pneumonia are available. Treatment depends on the underlying cause of bacterial pneumonia being treated with antibiotics.

The prognosis depends on the type of pneumonia, the treatment, any complications, and the person's underlying health. Pneumonia is a common disease that occurs in all age groups. It is a leading cause of death among the young, the old, and the chronically ill.

Signs and symptoms

People with infectious pneumonia often have a productive cough, fever accompanied by shaking chills, shortness of breath, sharp or stabbing chest pain during deep breaths, confusion, and an increased respiratory rate. In the elderly confusion may be the most prominent symptom. The typical symptoms in children under five are fever, cough, and fast or difficult breathing. Fever, however, is not very specific as it occurs in many other common illnesses and may be absent in those with severe disease or malnutrition while cough is frequently absent in those less than 2 months of age More severe symptoms may include central cyanosis, decreased drinking, convulsions, persistent vomiting, or a decreased level of consciousness.

Some causes of pneumonia are associated with specific symptoms. Pneumonia caused by *Legionella* may occur with abdominal pain and diarrhea, while pneumonia caused by tuberculosis or *Pneumocystis* may cause only weight loss and night sweats.

Physical examination may sometimes reveal low blood pressure, a high heart rate, or low oxygen saturation. Struggling to breathe, confusion and blue-tinged skin are signs of a medical emergency.

Findings from physical examination of the lungs may be normal, but often show decreased expansion of the chest on the affected side. Harsher sounds from the larger airways transmitted through the inflamed lung are heard as bronchial breathing on auscultation with a stethoscope. Rales (or crackles) may be heard over the affected area during inspiration. Percussion may be dulled over the affected lung, and increased rather than decreased vocal resonance distinguishes pneumonia from a pleural effusion.

Cause

Pneumonia can be due to microorganisms, irritants or unknown causes with infectious causes being the most common. Although more than one hundred strains of microorganism can cause pneumonia, only a few are responsible for most cases. The most common infectious causes are viruses and bacteria with less common being fungi and parasites. Mixed infections with both viruses and bacterial may occur in up to 45% of infections in children and 15% of infections in adults.

Viruses

In adults' viruses account for approximately a third of pneumonia cases. Commonly implicated agents include: rhinoviruses coronaviruses, influenza virus, respiratory syncytial virus (RSV), adenovirus, and parainfluenza Herpes simplex virus is a rare cause of pneumonia except in newborns. People with weakened immune systems are at increased risk of pneumonia caused by cytomegalovirus (CMV).

Bacteria

Bacteria are the most common cause of community acquired pneumonia with *Streptococcus pneumoniae* isolated in nearly 50%. Other commonly isolated bacteria include:*Haemophilus influenzae* in 20%, *Chlamydophila pneumoniae* in 13%,and Mycoplasma pneumoniae in 3%.

Other important Gram-positive cause of pneumonia is *Staphylococcus aureus*, with *Streptococcus agalactiae* being an important cause of pneumonia in newborn babies. Gram-negative bacteria cause pneumonia less frequently than gram-positive bacteria. Some of the gram-negative bacteria that cause pneumonia include *Hemophilus influenzae, Klebsiella pneumoniae, Escherichiacoli,Pseudomonas aeruginosa* and *Moraxella catarrhalis*. These bacteria often live in the stomach or intestines and may enter the lungs if vomit is inhaled. "Atypical" bacteria which because pneumonia include *Chlamydophila pneumoniae, Mycoplasma pneumoniae,* and *Legionella pneumophila*.

Fungi

Fungal pneumonia is uncommon, but it may occur in individuals with immune system problems due to AIDS, immunosuppressive drugs, or other medical problems. The pathophysiology of pneumonia caused by fungi is similar to that of bacterial pneumonia. Fungal pneumonia is most often caused by *Histoplasma capsulatum,* Blastomyces, *Cryptococcus neoformans, Pneumocystis jiroveci,* and *Coccidioides immitis*.

Parasites

A variety of parasites can affect the lungs. These parasites typically enter the body through the skin or by being swallowed. Once inside, they travel to the lungs, usually through the blood. There, as in other cases of pneumonia, a combination of cellular destruction and immune response causes disruption of oxygen transportation. One type of white blood cell, the eosinophil, responds vigorously to parasite infection. Eosinophils in the lungs can lead to eosinophilic pneumonia, thus complicating the underlying parasitic pneumonia. The most common parasites causing pneumonia are *Toxoplasma gondii, Strongyloidiasis stercoral is,* and *Ascariasis*.

Idiopathic

Idiopathic interstitial pneumonia or noninfectious pneumonia are a class of diffuse lung diseases. They include: diffuse alveolar damage, organizing pneumonia, nonspecific interstitial pneumonia, lymphocytic interstitial pneumonia, desquamative interstitial pneumonia, respiratory bronchiolitis interstitial lung disease, and usual interstitial pneumonia.

Pathophysiology

Viral

Viruses invade cells in order to reproduce. Typically, a virus reaches the lungs when airborne droplets are inhaled through the mouth and nose. Once in the lungs, the virus invades the cells lining the airways and alveoli. This invasion often leads to cell death, either when the virus directly kills the cells, or through a type of cell-controlled self-destruction called apoptosis. When the immune system responds to the viral infection, even more, lung damage occurs. White blood cells, mainly lymphocytes, activate certain chemical cytokines which allow fluid to leak into the alveoli. This combination of cell destruction and fluid-filled alveoli interrupts the normal transportation of oxygen into the bloodstream.

As well as damaging the lungs, many viruses affect other organs and thus disrupt many body functions. Viruses can also make the body more susceptible to bacterial infections; for which reason bacterial pneumonia may complicate viral pneumonia.

Bacterial

Bacteria typically enter the lung when airborne droplets are inhaled, but can also reach the lung through the bloodstream when there is an infection in another part of the body. Many bacteria live in parts of the upper respiratory tract, such as the nose, mouth and sinuses, and can easily be inhaled into the alveoli. Once inside, bacteria may invade the spaces between cells and between alveoli through connecting pores. This invasion triggers the immune system to send neutrophils, a type of defensive white blood cell, to the lungs. The neutrophils engulf and kill the offending organisms, and also release cytokines, causing a general activation of the immune system. This leads to the fever, chills, and fatigue common in bacterial and fungal pneumonia. The neutrophils, bacteria, and fluid from surrounding blood vessels fill the alveoli and interrupt normal oxygen transportation.

Diagnosis

Pneumonia is typically diagnosed based on a combination of physical signs and a chest X-ray. Confirming the underlying cause can be difficult however with no definitive test able to distinguish between bacterial and not bacterial aetiology. The World Health Organization has defined pneumonia in children clinical based on either a cough or difficulty breathing and a rapid respiratory rate, chest indrawing, or a decreased level of consciousness. A rapid respiratory rate is defined as greater than 50 breaths per minute in children two months to one year of age or greater than 40 breaths per minute in children one to five years of age. n those under two months of age a respiratory rate of greater than 60 per minute can be used. In children, an increased respiratory rate and lower chest indrawing are more sensitive than auscultation of chest crackles. Investigations are generally not needed in those with mild disease in those requiring admission to hospital pulse oximetry, chest radiography, and blood tests including a complete blood count, serum electrolytes, C-reactive protein, and possibly liver function tests are recommended.

Classification

Pneumonia can be classified in several ways. It is most commonly classified by where or how it was acquired (community-acquired, aspiration, healthcare-associated, hospital-acquired, and ventilator-associated pneumonia), but may also be classified by the area of the lung affected (lobar pneumonia, bronchial pneumonia and acute interstitial pneumonia) or by the causative organism Pneumonia in children may additionally be classified based on signs and symptoms into non-severe, severe, and very severe.

Imaging

A chest radiograph is frequently used in diagnosis. In people with the mild disease, it is recommended that imaging be restricted to those with potential complications, those who have not improved with treatment, or those in which the cause is uncertain. If a person, however, is sufficiently sick to require hospitalization a chest radiograph is recommended. Finding, however, does not always correlate with severity of disease and do not reliably distinguish between bacterial versus viral infection.

Xray signs of bacterial community-acquired pneumonia are classically lung consolidation of one lung segmental lobe Radiographic finding, however, may be variable especially in other types of pneumonia. Aspiration pneumonia may present with bilateral opacities primarily in the basis of the lungs and on the right side. While viral pneumonia may appear normal, be hyper-inflated, have patchy areas on both sides, or present similar to bacterial pneumonia with lobar consolidation. A CT scan can give additional information in indeterminate cases.

Microbiology

For people managed in the community figuring out the causative agent is not cost-effective and typically does not alter management for those who do not respond to treatment sputum culture should be considered and culture for *Mycobacterium tuberculosis* should be carried out in those with a chronic productive cough. Testing for other specific organisms may be recommended during outbreaks for public health reasons. In those who are hospitalized for severe disease both sputum and blood cultures are recommended. Viral infections can be confirmed via detection of either the virus or its antigens with culture or polymerase chain reaction (PCR) among other techniques. With routine microbiological testing a causative agent is determined in only 15% of cases.[9]

Differential diagnosis

Several diseases can present similar to pneumonia including: chronic obstructive pulmonary disease (COPD), asthma, pulmonary edema, bronchiectasis, lung cancer and pulmonary emboli. sects that can help distinguish these from pneumonia include the fact that COPD and asthma typically present with wheezing, pulmonary edema an abnormal electrocardiogram, bronchiectasis and lung cancer a cough of greater duration, and pulmonary emboli with acute onset sharp chest pain and shortness of breath.

Prevention

Prevention includes vaccination, environmental measures, and appropriately treating other diseases.

Vaccination

Vaccination is effective for preventing certain bacterial and viral pneumonia in both children and adults.

Influenza vaccines are modestly effective against influenza A and B the Center for Disease Control and Prevention (CDC) recommends that everyone 6 months and older get yearly vaccination. When an influenza outbreak is occurring, medications such as amantadine, rimantadine, zanamivir, and oseltamivir can help prevent influenza. Vaccinations against *Hemophilus influenzae* and *Streptococcus pneumoniae* in the first year of life have greatly reduced the role these bacteria play in causing pneumonia in children. Vaccinating children against *Streptococcus pneumoniae* has also led to a decreased incidence of these infections in adults because many adults acquire infections from children. Hib vaccine is now widely used around the globe. The childhood pneumococcal vaccine is still as of 2009 predominantly used in high-income countries, though this is changing. A vaccine against *Streptococcus pneumoniae* is also available for adults. It has been found to decrease the risk of invasive pneumococcal disease.

Environmental

Reducing indoor air pollution is recommended Smoking cessation is important not only because it helps to limit lung damage, but also, because cigarette smoke interferes with many of the body's natural defenses against pneumonia.

Other

Appropriately treating underlying illnesses (such as AIDS) can decrease a person's risk of pneumonia.

There are several ways to prevent pneumonia in newborn infants. Testing pregnant women for Group B Streptococcus and *Chlamydia trachomatis*, and then giving antibiotic treatment if needed, reduces pneumonia in infants. Suctioning the mouth and throat of infants with meconium-stained amniotic fluid decreases the rate of aspiration pneumonia.

Management

Typically, oral antibiotics, rest, and fluids are sufficient for complete resolution. However, people who are having trouble breathing, with other medical problems, and the elderly may need greater care. If the symptoms get worse, the pneumonia does not improve with home treatment, or complications occur, then hospitalization may be recommended. Over the counter cough medicine has not been found to be helpful in pneumonia Worldwide approximately 7-13% of cases in children result in hospitalization.

Bacterial

Antibiotics improve outcomes in those with bacterial pneumonia. Initially antibiotic choice depends on the characteristics of the person affected such as age, underlying health, and location the infection was acquired. In the UK empiric treatment is usually with amoxicillin, erythromycin, or azithromycin for community-acquired pneumonia. In North America, where the "atypical" forms of community-acquired pneumonia is becoming more common, macrolides (such as azithromycin), and doxycycline have displaced amoxicillin as first-line outpatient treatment the use of fluoroquinolones in uncomplicated cases is discouraged due to concerns of side effects and resistance. The duration of treatment has traditionally been seven to ten days, but there is increasing evidence that short courses (three to five days) are equivalent. Antibiotics recommended for hospital-acquired pneumonia include third- and fourth-generation cephalosporins, carbapenems, fluoroquinolones, aminoglycosides, and vancomycin These antibiotics are often given intravenously and may be used in combination.

Viral

Neuraminidase inhibitors may be used to treat viral pneumonia caused by influenza viruses (influenza A and influenza B). otherwise, no specific antiviral medication is recommended for other types of community-acquired pneumonia including SARS coronavirus, adenovirus, hantavirus, and parainfluenza virus. Influenza A may be treated with rimantadine or amantadine while influenza A or B may be treated with oseltamivir, zanamivir or peramivir. These are of most benefit if they are started within 48 hours of the onset of symptoms. Many strains of H5N1 influenza A, also known as avian influenza or "bird flu," have shown resistance to rimantadine and amantadine.

Aspiration

There is no evidence to support the use of antibiotics in chemical pneumonitis without bacterial superinfection. If the infection is present inspiration pneumonia, the choice of antibiotic will depend on several factors, including the suspected causative organism and whether pneumonia was acquired in the community or developed in a hospital setting. Common options include clindamycin, a combination of a beta-lactam antibiotic and metronidazole, or an aminoglycoside. Corticosteroids are commonly used in aspiration pneumonia, but there is no evidence to support their use either.

Prognosis

With treatment, most types of bacterial pneumonia can be cleared within two to four weeks and mortality is very low. Viral pneumonia may last longer, and mycoplasma pneumonia may take four to six weeks to resolve completely.

The most important complications include respiratory and circulatory failure and pleural effusions, empyema or abscesses.

Clinical prediction rules

Clinical prediction rules have been developed to more objectively prognosticate outcomes in pneumonia. Although these rules are often used in deciding whether or not to hospitalize the person, they were derived simply to inform on prognosis; neither index was designed or tested as guide to determine whether the person would benefit by hospital admission.

Pleural effusion, empyema, and abscess

In pneumonia, a collection of fluid (pleural effusion) often forms in the space that surrounds the lung (the pleural cavity).

Occasionally, microorganisms will infect this fluid thereby causing what is called an empyema. To distinguish an empyema from the more common simple parapneumonic effusion, the fluid is collected with a needle (thoracentesis) and examined. If this shows evidence of empyema, complete drainage of the fluid may be necessary, often requiring a chest tube. In severe cases of empyema, surgery may be needed. If the infected fluid is not drained, the infection may persist, because antibiotics do not penetrate well into the pleural cavity. If the fluid is sterile, it would only need drainage if very large, causing symptoms, or not resolving.

Rarely, bacteria in the lung will form a pocket of infected fluid called a lung abscess. Lung abscesses can usually be seen with a chest x-ray or chest CT scan. Abscesses typically occur inspiration pneumonia and often contain several types of bacteria.

Antibiotics are usually adequate to treat a lung abscess, but sometimes the abscess must be drained by a surgeon or radiologist.

Respiratory and circulatory failure

Because pneumonia affects the lungs, often people with pneumonia have difficulty breathing, and it may not be possible for them to breathe well enough to stay alive without support. Non-invasive breathing assistance may be helpful, such as with a bi-level positive airway pressure machine.

Pneumonia can also cause respiratory failure by triggering acute respiratory distress syndrome (ARDS), which results from a combination of infection and inflammatory response. The lungs quickly fill with fluid and become very stiff. This stiffness, combined with severe difficulties extracting oxygen due to the alveolar fluid, create a need for mechanical ventilation.

Sepsis and septic shock are potential complications of pneumonia. Sepsis occurs when microorganisms enter the bloodstream and the immune system responds by secreting cytokines. Sepsis most often occurs with bacterial pneumonia; *Streptococcus pneumoniae* is the most common cause. Individuals with sepsis or septic shock need hospitalization in an intensive care unit. They often require intravenous fluids and medications to help keep their blood pressure from dropping too low. Sepsis can cause liver,kidney, and heart damage, among other problems, and it often causes death.

CHAPTER NINE

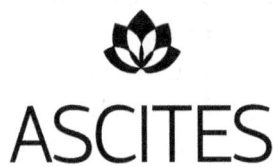

ASCITES

Ascites is a gastroenterological term for an accumulation of fluid in the peritoneal cavity. The medical condition is also known as peritoneal cavity fluid, peritoneal fluid excess, hydroperitoneum or more archaically as abdominal dropsy. Although most commonly due to cirrhosis and severe liver disease, its presence can portend other significant medical problems. Diagnosis of the cause is usually with blood tests, an ultrasound scan of the abdomen, and direct removal of the fluid by needle or paracentesis (which may also be therapeutic). Treatment may be with medication (diuretics), paracentesis, or other treatments directed at the cause.

Signs and symptoms

Mild ascites is hard to notice, but severe ascites leads to abdominal distension. Patients with ascites generally will complain of progressive abdominal heaviness and pressure as well as shortness of breath due to mechanical impingement on the diaphragm.

Ascites is detected on physical examination of the abdomen by visible bulging of the flanks in the reclining patient ("flank bulging"), "shifting dullness" (difference in percussion note in the flanks that shifts when the patient is turned on the side) or in massive ascites with a "fluid thrill" or "fluid wave" (tapping or pushing on one side will generate a wave-like effect through the fluid that can be felt in the opposite side of the abdomen).

Other signs of ascites may be present due to its underlying etiology. For instance, in portal hypertension (perhaps due to cirrhosis or fibrosis of the liver) patients may also complain of leg swelling, bruising, gynecomastia, hematemesis, or mental changes due to encephalopathy. Those with ascites due to cancer (peritoneal carcinomatosis) may complain of chronic fatigue or weight loss. Those with ascites due to heart failure may also complain of shortness of breath as well as wheezing and exercise intolerance.

Classification

Ascites exists in three grades:
- Grade 1: mild, only visible on ultrasound and CT
- Grade 2: detectable with flank bulging and shifting dullness
- Grade 3: directly visible, confirmed with fluid thrill

Diagnosis

Routine complete blood count (CBC), basic metabolic profile, liver enzymes, and coagulation should be performed. Most experts recommend a diagnostic paracentesis be performed if the ascites is new or if the patient with ascites is being admitted to the hospital. The fluid is then reviewed for its gross appearance, protein level, albumin, and cell counts (red and white). Additional tests will be performed if indicated such as Gram stain and cytopathology.

The *Serum-ascites albumin gradient* (SAAG) is probably a better discriminant than older measures (transudate versus exudate) for the causes of ascites. A high gradient (> 1.1 g/dL) indicates the ascites is due to portal hypertension. A low gradient (< 1.1 g/dL) indicates ascites of non-portal hypertensive etiology.

Ultrasound investigation is often performed prior to attempts to remove fluid from the abdomen. This may reveal the size and shape of the abdominal organs, and Doppler studies may show the direction of flow in the portal vein, as well as detecting Budd-Chiari syndrome and portal vein thrombosis. Additionally, the sonographer can make an estimation of the amount of ascitic fluid, and difficult-to-drain ascites may be drained under ultrasound guidance. Abdominal CT scan is a more accurate alternate to reveal abdominal organ structure and morphology.

Causes

Causes of high SAAG ("transudate") are: Cirrhosis - 81% (alcoholic in 65%, viral in 10%, cryptogenic in 6%)
- Heart failure - 3%
- Constrictive pericarditis
- Kwashiorkor
- Causes of low SAAG ("exudate") are:
- Cancer (primary peritoneal carcinomatosis and metastasis) - 10%
- Infection: Tuberculosis - 2% or Spontaneous bacterial peritonitis
- Pancreatitis - 1%
- Serositis

Pathophysiology

Ascitic fluid can accumulate as a transudate or an exudate. Amounts of up to 25 liters are possible.

Regardless of the cause, sequestration of fluid within the abdomen leads to additional fluid retention by the kidneys due to stimulatory effect on blood pressure hormones, notably aldosterone. The sympathetic nervous system is also activated, and renin production is increased due to decreased perfusion of the kidney. Extreme disruption of the renal blood flow can lead to hepatorenal syndrome. Other complications of ascites include spontaneous bacterial peritonitis (SBP), due to decreased antibacterial factors in the ascitic fluid such as complement.

Treatment

Ascites is generally treated while an underlying etiology is sought, in order to prevent complications, relieve symptoms, and prevent further progression. In patients with mild ascites, therapy is usually as an outpatient. The goal is weight loss of no more than kg/day for patients with both ascites and peripheral edema and no more than 0.5 kg/day for patients with ascites alone. In those with severe ascites causing a tense abdomen, hospitalization is generally necessary for paracentesis.

High SAAG

Treatments in high SAAG ("transudate") are:

Salt restriction

Salt restriction is the initial treatment, which allows diuresis (production of urine) since the patient now has more fluid than salt concentration. Salt restriction is effective in about 15% of patients.

Diuretics

Since salt restriction is the basic concept in treatment, and aldosterone is one of the hormones that acts to increase salt retention, a medication that counteracts aldosterone should be sought. Spironolactone (or other distal-tubule diuretics such

as triamterene or amiloride) is the drug of choice since they block the aldosterone receptor in the collecting tubule. Serum potassium level and renal function should be monitored closely while on these medications.

Monitoring diuresis: Diuresis can be monitored by weighing the patient daily. The goal is weight loss of no more than 1.0 kg/day for patients with both ascites and peripheral edema and no more than 0.5 kg/day for patients with ascites alone. A random urine sodium-to-potassium ratio of > 1 is 90% sensitivity in predicting negative balance (> 78-mmol/day sodium excretion).

Diuretic resistance: If a patient exhibits a resistance to or poor response to diuretic

therapy, ultrafiltration or aqua pheresis may be needed to achieve adequate control of fluid retention and congestion. The use of such mechanical methods of fluid removal can produce meaningful clinical benefits in patients with diuretic resistance and may restore responsiveness to conventional doses of diuretics.

Water restriction

Water restriction is needed if hyponatremia < 130 mmol per liter develops.

Paracentesis

In those with severe (tense) ascites, therapeutic paracentesis may be needed in addition to medical treatments listed above. As this may deplete serum albumin levels in the blood, albumin is generally administered intravenously in proportion to the amount of ascites removed.

Liver transplantation

Ascites that is refractory to medical therapy is considered an indication for liver transplantation. In the United States, the MELD score (online calculator) is used to prioritize patients for transplantation.

Shunting

In a minority of patients with advanced cirrhosis that have recurrent ascites, shunts may be used. Typical shunts used are portacaval shunt, peritoneovenous shunt, and the trans jugular intrahepatic portosystemic shunt (TIPS).

Low SAAG

Exudative ascites generally does not respond to manipulation of the salt balance or diuretic therapy. Repeated paracentesis and treatment of the underlying cause is the mainstay of treatment.

Complications

Spontaneous bacterial peritonitis Thrombosis

Complications involve portal vein thrombosis and splenic vein thrombosis: clotting of blood affects the hepatic portal vein or varices associated with splenic vein. Cirrhosis is a consequence of chronic liver disease characterized by replacement of liver tissue by fibrosis, scar tissue and regenerative nodules (lumps that occur as a result of a process in which damaged tissue is regenerated), leading to loss of liver function. Cirrhosis is most commonly caused by alcoholism, hepatitis B and C, and fatty liver disease, but has many other possible causes.

Ascites (fluid retention in the abdominal cavity) is the most common complication of cirrhosis, and is associated with a poor quality of life, increased risk of infection, and a poor long-term outcome. Other potentially life-threatening complications are hepatic encephalopathy (confusion and coma) and bleeding from esophageal varices.

Cirrhosis is generally irreversible, and treatment usually focuses on preventing progression and complications. In advanced stages of cirrhosis, the only option is a liver transplant.

The word "cirrhosis" derives from Greek word *cirrhosis* meaning *yellowish,*

tawny (the orange-yellow color of the diseased liver) + While the clinical entity was known before, it was René Laennec who gave it the name "cirrhosis" in his 1819.

Signs and symptoms

Some of the following signs and symptoms *may* occur in the presence of cirrhosis or as a result of the complications of cirrhosis. Many are nonspecific and may occur in other diseases and do not necessarily point to cirrhosis. Likewise, the absence of any does not rule out the possibility of cirrhosis.

Spider angiomata or *spider nevi*. Vascular lesions consisting of a central arteriole surrounded by many smaller vessels because of an increase in estradiol. These occur in about 1/3 of cases.

Palmar erythema. Exaggerations of normal speckled mottling of the palm, because of altered sex hormone metabolism.

Nail changes.

Muehrcke's lines - paired horizontal bands separated by normal color resulting from hypoalbuminemia (inadequate production of albumin).

Terry's nails - proximal two-thirds of the nail plate appears white with distal one-third red, also due to hypoalbuminemia

Clubbing - angle between the nail plate and proximal nail fold > 180 degrees

Hypertrophic osteoarthropathy. Chronic proliferative periostitis of the long bones that can cause considerable pain.

Dupuytren's contracture. Thickening and shortening of palmar fascia that leads to flexion deformities of the fingers. Thought to be caused by fibroblastic proliferation and disorderly collagen deposition. It is relatively common (33% of patients).

Gynecomastia. Benign proliferation of glandular tissue of male breasts presenting with a rubbery or firm mass extending concentrically from the nipples. This is caused by increased estradiol and can occur in up to 66% of patients.

Hypogonadism. Manifested as impotence, infertility, loss of sexual drive, and testicular atrophy because of primary gonadal injury or suppression of hypothalamic or pituitary function.

Liver size. Can be enlarged, normal, or shrunken.

Splenomegaly (increase in size of the spleen). Caused by congestion of the red pulp as a result of portal hypertension.

Ascites. Accumulation of fluid in the peritoneal cavity giving rise to flank dullness (needs about 1500 mL to detect flank dullness).

Caput medusa. In portal hypertension, the umbilical vein may open. Blood from the portal venous system may be shunted through the periumbilical veins into the umbilical vein and ultimately to the abdominal wall veins, manifesting as caput medusa.

Cruveilhier-Baumgarten murmur. Venous hum heard in epigastric region (on examination by stethoscope) because of collateral connections between portal system and the remnant of the umbilical vein in portal hypertension.

Fetor hepaticus. Musty odor in breath as a result of increased dimethyl sulfide.

Jaundice. Yellow discoloring of the skin, eye, and mucus membranes because of increased bilirubin (at least 2–3 mg/dL or 30 mmol/L). Urine may also appear dark.

Asterixis. Bilateral asynchronous flapping of outstretched, dorsiflexed hands seen in patients with hepatic encephalopathy.

Other. Weakness, fatigue, anorexia, weight loss.

Complications

As the disease progresses, complications may develop. In some people, these may be the first signs of the disease.

Bruising and bleeding resulting from decreased production of coagulation factors.

Jaundice as a result of decreased processing of bilirubin.

Itching (pruritus) because of bile salt products deposited in the skin.

Hepatic encephalopathy - the liver does not clear ammonia and related nitrogenous substances from the blood, which are carried to the brain, affecting cerebral functioning: neglect of personal appearance, unresponsiveness, forgetfulness, trouble concentrating, or changes in sleep habits.

Sensitivity to medication caused by decreased metabolism of the active compounds.

Hepatocellular carcinoma is primary liver cancer, a frequent complication of cirrhosis. It has a high mortality rate.

Portal hypertension - blood normally carried from the intestines and spleen through the hepatic portal vein flows more slowly and the pressure increases; this leads to the following complications:

Ascites - fluid leaks through the vasculature into the abdominal cavity.

Esophageal varices - collateral portal blood flow through vessels in the stomach and esophagus. These blood vessels may become enlarged and are more likely to burst.

Problems in other organs.

Cirrhosis can cause immune system dysfunction, leading to infection. Signs and symptoms of infection may be a specific are more difficult to recognize (e.g., worsening encephalopathy but no fever).

Fluid in the abdomen (ascites) may become infected with bacteria normally present in the intestines (spontaneous bacterial peritonitis).

Hepatorenal syndrome - insufficient blood supply to the kidneys, causing acute renal failure. This complication has a very high mortality (over 50%).

Hepatopulmonary syndrome - blood bypassing the normal lung circulation (shunting), leading to cyanosis and dyspnea (shortness of breath), characteristically worse on sitting up.

Porto pulmonary hypertension - increased blood pressure over the lungs as a consequence of portal hypertension.

Portal hypertensive gastropathy which refers to changes in the mucosa of the stomach in patients with portal hypertension, and is associated with cirrhosis severity.

Causes

Cirrhosis has many possible causes; sometimes more than one cause is present in the same patient. In the Western World, chronic alcoholism and hepatitis C are the most common causes.

Alcoholic liver disease (ALD). Alcoholic cirrhosis develops for between 10% and 20% of individuals who drink heavily for a decade or more. Alcohol seems to injure the liver by blocking the normal metabolism of protein, fats, and carbohydrates. Patients may also have concurrent alcoholic hepatitis with fever, hepatomegaly, jaundice, and anorexia. AST and ALT are both elevated but less than 300 IU/L with an AST:ALT ratio > 2.0, a value rarely seen in other liver diseases. Liver biopsy may show hepatocyte necrosis, Mallory bodies, neutrophilic infiltration with perivenular inflammation.

Non-alcoholic steatohepatitis (NASH). In NASH, fat builds up in the liver and eventually causes scar tissue. This type of hepatitis appears to be associated with diabetes, protein malnutrition, obesity, coronary artery disease, and treatment with corticosteroid medications. This disorder is similar to that of alcoholic liver disease but patient does not have an alcohol history. Biopsy is needed for diagnosis.

Chronic hepatitis C. Infection with the hepatitis C virus causes inflammation of the liver and a variable grade of damage to the organ that over several decades can lead to cirrhosis. Cirrhosis caused by hepatitis C is the most common reason for liver transplant. Can be diagnosed with serologic assays that detect hepatitis C antibody or viral RNA. The enzyme immunoassay, EIA-2, is the most commonly used screening test in the US.

Chronic hepatitis B. The hepatitis B virus causes liver inflammation and injury that over several decades can lead to cirrhosis. Hepatitis D is dependent on the presence of hepatitis B and accelerates cirrhosis in co-infection. Chronic hepatitis B can be diagnosed with detection of HBsAG > 6 months after initial infection. HBeAG and

HBV DNA are determined to assess whether patient will need antiviral therapy.

Primary biliary cirrhosis. May be asymptomatic or complain of fatigue, pruritus, and non-jaundice skin hyperpigmentation with hepatomegaly. There is prominent alkaline phosphatase elevation as well as elevations in cholesterol and bilirubin. Gold standard diagnosis is antimitochondrial antibodies with liver biopsy as confirmation if showing florid bile duct lesions. It is more common in women.

Primary sclerosing cholangitis. PSC is a progressive cholestatic disorder presenting with pruritus, steatorrhea, fat soluble vitamin deficiencies, and metabolic bone disease. There is a strong association with inflammatory bowel disease (IBD), especially ulcerative colitis. Diagnosis is best with contrast cholangiography showing diffuse, multifocal strictures and focal dilation of bile ducts, leading to a beaded appearance. Non-specific serum immunoglobulins may also be elevated.

Autoimmune hepatitis. This disease is caused by the immunologic damage to the liver causing inflammation and eventually scarring and cirrhosis. Findings include elevations in serum globulins, especially gamma globulins. Therapy with prednisone and/or azathioprine is beneficial. Cirrhosis due to autoimmune hepatitis still has 10-year survival of 90%+. There is no specific tool to diagnose autoimmune but it can be beneficial to initiate a trial of corticosteroids.

Hereditary hemochromatosis. Usually presents with family history of cirrhosis, skin hyperpigmentation, diabetes mellitus, pseudogout, and/or cardiomyopathy, all due to signs of iron overload. Labs will show fasting transferrin saturation of > 60% and ferritin > 300 ng/mL. Genetic testing may be used to identify *HFE* mutations. If these are present, biopsy may not need to be performed. Treatment is with phlebotomy to lower total body iron levels.

Wilson's disease. Autosomal recessive disorder characterized by low serum ceruloplasmin and increased hepatic copper content on liver biopsy. May also have Kayser-Fleischer rings in the cornea and altered mental status.

Alpha 1-antitrypsin deficiency (AAT). Autosomal recessive disorder. Patients may also have COPD, especially if they have a history of tobacco smoking. Serum AAT levels are low. Recombinant AAT is used to prevent lung disease due to AAT deficiency.

Cardiac cirrhosis. Due to chronic right sided heart failure which leads to liver congestion.

Galactosemia

Glycogen storage disease type IV

Cystic fibrosis

Hepatotoxic drugs or toxins

Certain parasitic infections (such as schistosomiasis)

Lysosomal acid lipase deficiency (LAL Deficiency) is a rare autosomal recessive genetic condition and is characterized by hepatomegaly, persistently abnormal LFTs and type II hyperlipidemia. Splenomegaly and evidence of mild hypersplenism may affect some patients. Untreated, LAL Deficiency may lead to fibrosis, cirrhosis, liver failure and death.

Pathophysiology

The liver plays a vital role in synthesis of proteins (e.g., albumin, clotting factors and complement), detoxification and storage (e.g., vitamin A). In addition, it participates in the metabolism of lipids and carbohydrates.

Cirrhosis is often preceded by hepatitis and fatty liver (steatosis), independent of the cause. If the cause is removed at this stage, the changes are still fully reversible.

The pathological hallmark of cirrhosis is the development of scar tissue that replaces normal parenchyma, blocking the portal flow of blood through the organ and disturbing normal function.

The fibrous tissue bands (septa) separate hepatocyte nodules, which eventually replace the entire liver architecture, leading to decreased blood flow throughout. The spleen becomes congested, which leads to hypersplenism and increased sequestration of platelets. Portal hypertension is responsible for the most severe complications of cirrhosis.

Diagnosis

The gold standard for diagnosis of cirrhosis is a liver biopsy, through a percutaneous, transjugular, laparoscopic, or fine-needle approach. A biopsy is not necessary if the clinical, laboratory and radiologic data suggest cirrhosis.

Furthermore, there is a small but significant risk to liver biopsy, and cirrhosis itself predisposes for complications due to liver biopsy.

Lab findings

The following findings are typical in cirrhosis:

Aminotransferases - AST and ALT are moderately elevated, with AST > ALT. However, normal aminotransferases do not preclude cirrhosis.

Alkaline phosphatase - usually slightly elevated.

Gamma-glutamyl transferase – correlates with AP levels. Typically, much higher in chronic liver disease from alcohol.

Bilirubin - may elevate as cirrhosis progresses.

Albumin - levels fall as the synthetic function of the liver declines with worsening cirrhosis since albumin is exclusively synthesized in the liver

Prothrombin time - increases since the liver synthesizes clotting factors.

Globulins - increased due to shunting of bacterial antigens away from the liver to lymphoid tissue.

Serum sodium - hyponatremia due to inability to excrete free water resulting from high levels of ADH and aldosterone.

Thrombocytopenia - due to both congestive splenomegaly as well as

decreased thrombopoietin from the liver. However, this rarely results in platelet count < 50,000/mL.

Leukopenia and neutropenia - due to splenomegaly with splenic margination.

Coagulation defects - the liver produces most of the coagulation factors and thus coagulopathy correlates with worsening liver disease.

There is now a validated and patented combination of 6 of these markers as non- invasive biomarker of fibrosis (and so of cirrhosis): FibroTest.

Other laboratory studies performed in newly diagnosed cirrhosis may include:

Serology for hepatitis viruses, autoantibodies (ANA, anti-smooth muscle, anti- mitochondria, anti-LKM)

Ferritin and transferrin saturation (markers of iron

overload), copper and ceruloplasmin (markers of copper overload)

Immunoglobulin levels (IgG, IgM, IgA) - these are non-specific but may assist in distinguishing various causes

Cholesterol and glucose

Alpha 1-antitrypsin

Imaging

Ultrasound is routinely used in the evaluation of cirrhosis, where it may show a small and nodular liver in advanced cirrhosis along with increased echogenicity with irregular appearing areas. Ultrasound may also screen for hepatocellular carcinoma, portal hypertension and Budd-Chiari syndrome (by assessing flow in the hepatic vein).

A new type of device, the Fibro Scan (transient elastography), uses elastic waves to determine liver stiffness which theoretically can be converted into a liver score based on the METAVIR scale. The Fibro Scan produces an ultrasound image of the liver (from 20–80 mm) along with a pressure reading (in kPa.) The test is much faster than a biopsy (usually last 2.5–5 minutes) and is completely painless. It shows reasonable correlation with the severity of cirrhosis.

Other tests performed in particular circumstances include abdominal CT and liver/bile duct MRI (MRCP).

Endoscopy

Gastroscopy (endoscopic examination of the esophagus, stomach and duodenum) is performed in patients with established cirrhosis to exclude the possibility of esophageal varices. If these are found, prophylactic local therapy may be applied (sclerotherapy or banding) and beta-blocker treatment may be commenced.

Rarely diseases of the bile ducts, such as primary sclerosing cholangitis, can be causes of cirrhosis. Imaging of the bile ducts, such as ERCP or MRCP (MRI of biliary tract and pancreas) can show abnormalities in these patients, and may aid in the diagnosis.

Pathology

Macroscopically, the liver is initially enlarged, but with the progression of the disease, it becomes smaller. Its surface is irregular, the consistency is firm and the color is often yellow. Depending on the size of the nodules there are three macroscopic types: micronodular, macronodular and mixed cirrhosis. In micronodular form (Laennec's cirrhosis or portal cirrhosis) regenerating nodules are under 3 mm. In macronodular cirrhosis (post-necrotic cirrhosis), the nodules are larger than 3 mm.

The mixed cirrhosis consists of a variety of nodules with different sizes.

However, cirrhosis is defined by its pathological features on microscopy: (1) the presence of regenerating nodules of hepatocytes and (2) the presence of fibrosis, or the deposition of connective tissue between these nodules. The fibrosis in cirrhosis can lead to destruction of other normal tissues in the liver: including the sinusoids, the space of Disse, and other vascular structures, which leads to altered resistance to blood flow in the liver and portal hypertension.

Grading

The severity of cirrhosis is commonly classified with the Child-Pugh score. This score uses bilirubin, albumin, INR, presence and severity of ascites and encephalopathy to classify patients in class A, B or C; class A has a favorable prognosis, while class C is at high risk of death. It was devised in 1964 by Child and Turcotte and modified in 1973 by Pugh *et al.*

More modern scores, used in the allocation of liver transplants but also in other contexts, are the Model for End-Stage Liver Disease (MELD) score and its pediatric counterpart, the Pediatric End-Stage Liver Disease (PELD) score.

The hepatic venous pressure gradient, i.e., the difference in venous pressure between afferent and efferent blood to the liver, also determines the severity of cirrhosis, although hard to measure. A value of 16 mm or more means a greatly increased risk of dying.

Management

Generally, liver damage from cirrhosis cannot be reversed, but treatment could stop or delay further progression and reduce complications. A healthy diet is encouraged, as cirrhosis may be an energy-consuming process. Close follow-up is often necessary.

Antibiotics will be prescribed for infections, and various medications can help with itching. Laxatives, such as lactulose, decrease the risk of constipation; their role in preventing encephalopathy is limited.

Treating underlying causes

Alcoholic cirrhosis caused by alcohol abuse is treated by abstaining from alcohol. Treatment for hepatitis-related cirrhosis involves medications used to treat the different types of hepatitis, such as interferon for viral hepatitis and corticosteroids for autoimmune hepatitis. Cirrhosis caused by Wilson's disease, in which copper builds up in organs, is treated with chelation therapy (e.g., penicillamine) to remove the copper.

Preventing further liver damage

Regardless of underlying cause of cirrhosis, alcohol and paracetamol, as well as other potentially damaging substances, are discouraged. Vaccination of susceptible patients should be considered for Hepatitis A and Hepatitis B.

Preventing complications

Ascites

Salt restriction is often necessary, as cirrhosis leads to accumulation of salt (sodium retention). Diuretics may be necessary to suppress ascites.

Esophageal variceal bleeding

For portal hypertension, propranolol is a commonly used agent to lower blood pressure over the portal system. In severe complications from portal hypertension, transjugular intrahepatic portosystemic shunting is occasionally indicated to relieve pressure on the portal vein. As this can worsen encephalopathy, it is reserved for those at low risk of encephalopathy, and is generally regarded only as a bridge to liver transplantation or as a palliative measure.

Hepatic encephalopathy

High-protein food increases the nitrogen balance, and would theoretically
increase encephalopathy; in the past, this was therefore eliminated as much as possible from the diet. Recent studies show that this assumption was incorrect, and high- protein foods are even *encouraged* to maintain adequate nutrition.

Hepatorenal syndrome

The hepatorenal syndrome is defined as a urine sodium less than 10 mmol/L and
a serum creatinine > 1.5 mg/dl (or 24-hour creatinine clearance less than 40 ml/min) after a trial of volume expansion without diuretics.

Spontaneous bacterial peritonitis

Cirrhotic patients with ascites are at risk of spontaneous bacterial peritonitis.

Transplantation-

If complications cannot be controlled or when the liver ceases functioning, liver transplantation is necessary. Survival from liver transplantation has been improving over the 1990s, and the five-year survival rate is now around 80%, depending largely on the severity of disease and other medical problems in the recipient.

Decompensated cirrhosis

In patients with previously stable cirrhosis, decompensation may occur due to various causes, such as constipation, infection (of any source), increased alcohol
intake, medication, bleeding from esophageal varices or dehydration. It may take the form of any of the complications of cirrhosis listed above.

Patients with decompensated cirrhosis generally require admission to hospital, with close monitoring of the fluid balance, mental status, and emphasis on adequate nutrition and medical treatment - often with diuretics, antibiotics, laxatives and/or enemas, thiamine and
occasionally steroids, acetylcysteine and pentoxifylline. Administration of saline is generally avoided as it would add to the already high total body sodium content that typically occurs in cirrhosis.

CHAPTER TEN

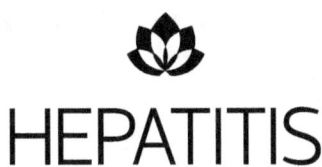

HEPATITIS

Hepatitis is defined by the inflammation of the liver and characterized by the presence of inflammatory cells in the tissue of the organ. The name is derived from the Greek *hepar,* the root being *hepat-* meaning *liver*, and suffix *-itis*, meaning "inflammation".

Hepatitis may occur with limited or no symptoms, but often leads to jaundice, anorexia (poor appetite) and malaise. Hepatitis is acute when it lasts less than six months and chronic when it persists longer. A group of viruses known as the hepatitis viruses cause most cases of hepatitis worldwide, but it can also be due to toxins (notably alcohol, certain medications, some industrial organic solvents and plants), other infections and autoimmune diseases.

Signs and symptoms

Acute

Initial features are of nonspecific flu-like symptoms, common to almost all acute viral infections and may include malaise, muscle and joint aches, fever, nausea or vomiting, diarrhea, and headache. More specific symptoms, which can be present in acute hepatitis from any cause, are: profound loss of appetite, aversion to smoking among smokers, dark urine, yellowing of the eyes and skin (i.e., jaundice) and abdominal discomfort. Physical findings are usually minimal, apart from jaundice in third and tender hepatomegaly (swelling of the liver) in about 10%. Some exhibit lymphadenopathy (enlarged lymph nodes, in 5%) or splenomegaly (enlargement of the spleen, in 5%).

Acute viral hepatitis is more likely to be asymptomatic in younger people. Symptomatic individuals may present after convalescent stage of 7 to 10 days, with the total illness lasting 2 to 6 weeks.

A small proportion of people with acute hepatitis progress to acute liver failure, in which t he liver is unable to clear harmful substances from the circulation (leading to confusion and coma due to hepatic encephalopathy) and produce blood proteins (leading to peripheral edema and bleeding). This may become life-threatening and occasionally requires a liver transplant.

Chronic

Chronic hepatitis often leads to nonspecific symptoms such as malaise, tiredness and weakness, and often leads to no symptoms at all. It is commonly identified on blood tests performed either for screening or to evaluate nonspecific symptoms. The occurrence of jaundice indicates advanced liver damage. On physical examination there may be enlargement of the liver

Extensive damage and scarring of liver (i.e. cirrhosis) leads to weight loss, easy bruising and bleeding tendencies, peripheral edema (swelling of the legs) and accumulation of ascites (fluid in the abdominal cavity). Eventually, cirrhosis may lead to various complications: esophageal varices (enlarged veins in the wall of the esophagus that can cause life-threatening bleeding) hepatic encephalopathy (confusion and coma) and hepatorenal syndrome (kidney dysfunction).

Acne, abnormal menstruation, lung scarring, inflammation of the thyroid gland and kidneys may be present in women with autoimmune hepatitis.

Causes

Acute-

Viral hepatitis:
    Hepatitis A, B, C, D, and E.
    Yellow fever
    adenoviruses
    Non-viral infection
    toxoplasma
    Leptospira
    Q fever
    rocky mountain spotted fever
    Alcohol
    Toxins: Amanita toxin in mushrooms, carbon tetrachloride, asafoetida
Drugs- Paracetamol, amoxycillin, antituberculosis medicines, minocycline and many others (see longer list below).
    Ischemic hepatitis (circulatory insufficiency)
    Pregnancy
    Auto immune conditions, e.g., Systemic Lupus Erythematosus (SLE)
    Metabolic diseases, e.g., Wilson's disease

Chronic-

    Viral hepatitis: Hepatitis B with or without hepatitis D, hepatitis C (neither hepatitis A nor hepatitis E causes chronic hepatitis)
    Autoimmune
    Autoimmune hepatitis
    Alcohol
    Drugs
    methyldopa
    nitrofurantoin
    isoniazid
    ketoconazole
    Non-alcoholic steatohepatitis
    Heredity
    Wilson's disease
    alpha 1-antitrypsin deficiency

Alcoholic hepatitis

Ethanol, mostly in alcoholic beverages, is a significant cause of hepatitis. Usually alcoholic hepatitis comes after a period of increased alcohol consumption. Alcoholic hepatitis is characterized by a variable constellation of symptoms, which may include feeling unwell, enlargement of the liver, development of fluid in the abdomen ascites, and modest elevation of liver blood tests. Alcoholic hepatitis can vary from mild with only liver test elevation to severe liver inflammation with development of jaundice, prolonged prothrombin time, and liver failure. Severe cases are characterized by either obtundation (dulled consciousness) or the combination of elevated bilirubin levels and prolonged prothrombin time; the mortality rate in both categories is 50% within 30 days of onset.

Alcoholic hepatitis is distinct from cirrhosis caused by long term alcohol consumption. Alcoholic hepatitis can occur in patients with chronic alcoholic liver disease and alcoholic cirrhosis. Alcoholic hepatitis by itself does not lead to cirrhosis, but cirrhosis is more common in patients with long term alcohol consumption. Patients who drink alcohol to excess are also more often than others found to have hepatitis C The combination of hepatitis C and alcohol consumption accelerates the development of cirrhosis.

Drug induced

A large number of drugs can cause hepatitis:

Agomelatine (antidepressant)

Allopurinol

Amitriptyline (antidepressant)

Paracetamol (acetaminophen in the United States) can cause hepatitis when taken in an overdose. The severity of liver damage may be limited by prompt administration of acetylcysteine.

Phenytoin and valproic acid (antiepileptics)

Troglitazone (antidiabetic, withdrawn in 2000 for causing hepatitis)

Zidovudine (antiretroviral i.e., against HIV)

Some herbs and nutritional supplements the clinical course of drug-induced hepatitis is quite variable, depending on the drug and the patient's tendency to react to the drug. For example, halothane hepatitis can range from mild to fatal as can INH-induced hepatitis. Hormonal contraception can cause structural changes in the liver. Amiodarone hepatitis can be untreatable since the long half-life of the drug (up to 60 days) means that there is no effective way to stop exposure to the drug. Statins can cause elevations of liver function blood tests normally without indicating an underlying hepatitis. Lastly, human variability is such that any drug can be a cause of hepatitis.

Other toxins

Other Toxins can cause hepatitis:

Amatoxin-containing mushrooms, including the Death Cap (*Amanita phalloides*), the Destroying

Angel (*Amanita ocreata*), and some species of *Galerina*. A portion of a single mushroom can be enough to be lethal (10 mg or less of α-amanitin).

White phosphorus, an industrial toxin and war chemical.

Carbon tetrachloride ("tetra", a dry-cleaning agent), chloroform, and trichloroethylene, all chlorinated hydrocarbons, cause steatohepatitis (hepatitis with fatty liver).

Metabolic disorders

Some metabolic disorders cause different forms of hepatitis. Hemochromatosis (due to iron accumulation) and Wilson's disease (copper accumulation) can cause liver inflammation and necrosis.

Non-alcoholic steatohepatitis (NASH) is effectively a consequence of metabolic syndrome.

Obstructive

"Obstructive jaundice" is the term used to describe jaundice due to obstruction of the bile duct (by gallstones or external obstruction by cancer). If longstanding, it leads to destruction and inflammation of liver tissue.

Autoimmune

Anomalous presentation of human leukocyte antigen (HLA) class II on the surface of hepatocytes, possibly due to genetic predisposition or acute liver infection; causes a cell-mediated immune response against the body's own liver, resulting in autoimmune hepatitis.

Alpha 1-antitrypsin deficiency

In severe cases of alpha 1-antitrypsin deficiency (A1AD), the accumulated protein in the endoplasmic reticulum causes liver cell damage and inflammation.

Non-alcoholic fatty liver disease

Non-alcoholic fatty liver disease (NAFLD) is the occurrence of fatty liver in people who have no history of alcohol use. It is most commonly associated with obesity (80% of all obese people have fatty liver). It is more common in women. Severe NAFLD leads to inflammation, a state referred to as *non-alcoholic steatohepatitis* (NASH), which on biopsy of the liver resembles alcoholic hepatitis (with fat droplets and inflammatory cells, but usually no Mallory bodies).

The diagnosis depends on medical history, physical exam, blood tests, radiological imaging and sometimes a liver biopsy. The initial evaluation to identify the presence of fatty infiltration of the liver is medical imaging,

including such ultrasound, computed tomography (CT), or magnetic resonance (MRI). However, imaging cannot readily identify inflammation in the liver. Therefore, the differentiation between steatosis and NASH often requires a liver biopsy. It can also be difficult to distinguish NASH from alcoholic hepatitis when the patient has a history of alcohol consumption. Sometimes in such cases a trial of abstinence from alcohol along with follow- up blood tests and a repeated liver biopsy are required.

NASH is becoming recognized as the most important cause of liver disease second only to hepatitis C in numbers of patients going on to cirrhosis

Ischemic hepatitis

Ischemic hepatitis is caused by decreased circulation to the liver cells. Usually this is due to decreased blood pressure (or shock), leading to the equivalent term "shock liver". Patients with ischemic hepatitis are usually very ill due to the underlying cause of shock. Rarely, ischemic hepatitis can be caused by local problems with the blood vessels that supply oxygen to the liver (such as thrombosis, or clotting of the hepatic artery which partially supplies blood to liver cells). Blood testing of a person with ischemic hepatitis will show very high levels of transaminase enzymes (AST and ALT), which may exceed 1000 U/L. The elevation in these blood tests is usually transient (lasting 7 to 10 days). It is rare that liver function will be affected by ischemic hepatitis.

CHAPTER ELEVEN

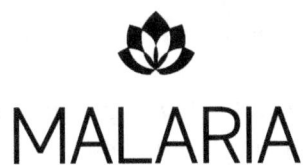

MALARIA

Malaria in humans is caused by eukaryotic protists of the genus *Plasmodium*. It is widespread in tropical and subtropical regions, including much of Sub-Saharan Africa, Asia and the Americas. Malaria is very prevalent in these regions because they have significant amounts of rainfall and consistently hot temperatures. These warm, consistent temperatures and moisture provide mosquitos with the environment they need to breed continuously. The cause of the disease is a protozoan, discovered in 1880, by Charles Louis Alphonse Laveran while he was working in the military hospital in Constantine, Algeria and observed the parasites in a blood smear taken from a patient who had just died of malaria. The disease results from the multiplication of malaria parasites within red blood cells, causing symptoms that typically include fever and headache, in severe cases progressing to coma, and death.

Four species of *Plasmodium* can infect and be transmitted by humans. Severe disease is largely caused by *Plasmodium falciparum*. Malaria caused by *Plasmodiumvivax*, *Plasmodium oval* and *Plasmodium malariae* is generally a milder disease that is rarely fatal. A fifth species,*Plasmodium knowlesi*, is a zoonosis that causes malaria in macaques but can also infect humans. Malaria transmission can be reduced by preventing mosquito bites by distribution of inexpensive mosquito nets and insect repellents, or by mosquito-control measures such as spraying insecticides inside houses and draining standing water where mosquitoes lay their eggs. Although many are under development, the challenge of producing a widely available vaccine that provides a high level of protection for a sustained period is still to be met. Two drugs are also available to prevent malaria in travellers to malaria-endemic countries (prophylaxis).

A variety of antimalarial medications are available. In the last 5 years, treatment of *P. falciparum* infections in endemic countries has been transformed by the use of combinations of drugs containing an artemisinin derivative. Severe malaria is treated with intravenous or intramuscular quinine or, increasingly, the artemisinin derivative artesunate which is superior to quinine in both children and adults. Resistance has developed to several antimalarial drugs, most notably chloroquine.

Each year, there are more than 225 million cases of malaria, killing around 781,000 people each year according to the World Health Organization's 2010 World Malaria Report, 2.23% of deaths worldwide. The majority of deaths are of young children in sub-Saharan Africa. Ninety per cent of malaria-related deaths occur in sub-Saharan Africa. Malaria is commonly associated with poverty, and can indeed be a cause of poverty and a major hindrance to economic development.

Signs and symptoms

Typical fever patterns of malaria

symptoms of malaria include fever, shivering, arthralgia (joint pain), vomiting, anemia (caused by hemolysis), hemoglobinuria, retinal damage, and convulsions. The classic symptom of malaria is cyclical occurrence of sudden coldness followed by rigor and then fever and sweating lasting four to six hours, occurring every two days in *P. vivax* and *P. ovale* infections, while every three days for *P. malariae*. *P. falciparum* can have recurrent fever every 36–48 hours or a less pronounced and almost continuous fever. For reasons that are poorly understood, but that may be related to high intracranial pressure, children with malaria frequently exhibit abnormal posturing, a sign indicating severe brain damage. Malaria has been found to cause cognitive impairments, especially in children. It causes widespread anemia during a period of rapid brain development and also direct brain damage. This neurologic damage results from cerebral malaria to which children are more vulnerable Cerebral malaria is associated with retinal whitening, which may be a useful clinical sign in distinguishing malaria from other causes of fever.

Severe malaria is almost exclusively caused by *P. falciparum* infection, and usually arises 6–14 days after infection. Consequences of severe malaria include coma and death if untreated—young children and pregnant women are especially

vulnerable. Splenomegaly (enlarged spleen), severe headache,

cerebral ischemia, hepatomegaly (enlarged liver), hypoglycemia, and hemoglobinuria with renal failure may occur. Renal failure is a feature of blackwater fever, where hemoglobin from lysed red blood cells leaks into the urine. Severe malaria can progress extremely rapidly and cause death within hours or days. In the most severe cases of the

disease, fatality rates can exceed 20%, even with intensive care and treatment. In endemic areas, treatment is often less satisfactory and the overall fatality rate for all cases of malaria can be as high as one in ten. Over the longer term, developmental impairments have been documented in children who have suffered episodes of severe malaria.

Cause

A *Plasmodium* sporozoite traverses the cytoplasm of a mosquito midgut epithelial cell in this false-color electron micrograph.

Malaria parasites are members of the genus *Plasmodium* (phylum Apicomplexa). In human's malaria is caused by *P. falciparum, P. malariae, P. ovale, P. vivax* and *P. knowlesi. P. falciparum* is the most common cause of infection, and is also responsible for about 90% of the deaths from malaria. Parasitic *Plasmodium* species also infect birds, reptiles, monkeys, chimpanzees and rodents There have been documented human infections with several simian species of malaria, namely *P. knowlesi, P. inui, P. cynomolgi, P. simiovale, P. brazilianum, P. schwetzi* and *P. simium*; however, with the exception of *P. knowlesi*, these are mostly of limited public health importance.

Life cycle

The parasite's secondary (intermediate) hosts are humans and other vertebrates. Female mosquitoes of the *Anopheles* genus are primary hosts and transmission vectors. Young mosquitoes first ingest the malaria parasite by feeding on an infected human carrier and the infected *Anopheles* mosquitoes carry*Plasmodium* sporozoites in their salivary glands. A mosquito becomes infected when it takes a blood meal from an infected human. Once ingested, the parasite gametocytes taken up in the blood will further differentiate into male or female gametes and then fuse in the mosquito's gut. This produces an ookinete that penetrates the gut lining and produces an oocyst in the gut wall. When the oocyst ruptures, it releases sporozoites that migrate through the mosquito's body to the salivary glands, where they are then ready to infect a new human host. This type of transmission is occasionally referred to as anterior station transfer. The sporozoites are injected into the skin, alongside saliva, when the mosquito takes a subsequent blood meal.

Only female mosquitoes feed on blood while male mosquitoes feed on plant nectar, thus males do not transmit the disease. The females of the *Anopheles* genus of mosquito prefer to feed at night. They usually start searching for a meal at dusk, and will continue throughout the night until taking a meal. Malaria parasites can also be transmitted by blood transfusions, although this is rare.

Recurrent malaria

Malaria recurs after treatment for three reasons. Recrudescence occurs when parasites are not cleared by treatment, whereas reinfection indicates complete clearance with new infection established from a separate infective mosquito bite; both can occur with any malaria parasite species. Relapse is specific to *P. vivax* and *P. ovale* and involves re- emergence of blood-stage parasites from latent parasites (hypnozoites) in the liver.

Describing a case of malaria as cured by observing the disappearance of parasites from the bloodstream can, therefore, be deceptive. The longest incubation period reported for a *P. vivax* infection is 30 years. Approximately one in five of *P. vivax* malaria cases

in temperate areas involve overwintering by hypnozoites (i.e., relapses begin the year after the mosquito bite) The life cycle of malaria parasites in the human body. A mosquito infects a person by taking a blood meal. First, sporozoites enter the bloodstream and migrate to the liver. They infect liver cells (hepatocytes), where they multiply into merozoites, rupture the liver cells, and escape back into the bloodstream. Then, the merozoites infect red blood cells, where they develop into ring forms, trophozoites and schizonts which in turn produce further merozoites. Sexual forms (gametocytes) are also produced, which, if taken up by a mosquito, will infect the insect and continue the life cycle.

Pathogenesis

Malaria develops via two phases: an exoerythrocytic and an erythrocytic phase. The exoerythrocytic phase involves infection of the hepatic system, or liver, whereas the erythrocytic phase involves infection of the erythrocytes or red blood cells. When an infected mosquito pierces a person's skin to take a blood meal, sporozoites in the mosquito's saliva enter the bloodstream and migrate to the liver. Within minutes of being introduced into the human host, the sporozoites infect hepatocytes, multiplying asexually and asymptomatically for a period of 8–30 days. Once in the liver, these organisms differentiate to yield thousands of merozoites, which, following rupture of their host cells, escape into the blood and infect red blood cells, thus beginning the erythrocytic stage of the life cycle. The parasite escapes from the liver undetected by wrapping itself in the cell membrane of the infected host liver cell. Within the red blood cells, the parasites multiply further, again asexually, periodically breaking out of their hosts to invade fresh red blood cells. Several such amplification cycles occur. Thus, classical descriptions of waves of fever arise from simultaneous waves of merozoites escaping and infecting red blood cells.

Some *P. vivax* and *P. ovale* sporozoites do not immediately develop into exoerythrocytic- phase merozoites, but instead produce hypnozoites that remain dormant for periods ranging from several months (6–12 months is typical) to as long as three years. After a period of dormancy, they reactivate and produce merozoites. Hypnozoites are responsible for long incubation and late relapses in these two species of malaria.

The parasite is relatively protected from attack by the body's immune system because for most of its human life cycle it resides within the liver and blood cells and is relatively invisible to immune surveillance. However, circulating infected blood cells are destroyed in the spleen. To avoid this fate, the *P. falciparum* parasite displays adhesive proteins on the surface of the infected blood cells, causing the blood cells to stick to the walls of small blood vessels, thereby sequestering the parasite from passage through the general circulation and the spleen. This "stickiness" is the main factor giving rise to hemorrhagic complications of malaria. High endothelial venules (the smallest branches of the circulatory system) can be blocked by the attachment of masses of these infected red blood cells. The blockage of these vessels causes symptoms such as in placental and cerebral malaria. In cerebral malaria the sequestrated red blood cells can breach the blood brain barrier possibly leading to coma.

Although the red blood cell surface adhesive proteins (called PfEMP1, for *Plasmodium falciparum* erythrocyte membrane protein 1) are exposed to the immune system, they do not serve as good immune targets, because of their extreme diversity; there are at least 60 variations of the protein within a single parasite and effectively limitless versions within parasite populations. The parasite switches between a broad repertoire of PfEMP1 surface proteins, thus staying one step ahead of the pursuing immune system.

Some merozoites turn into male and female gametocytes. Since the gametocytes are formed in the blood of the vertebrate host, the vertebrate host is the definitive host of the disease. If a mosquito pierces the skin of an infected person, it potentially picks up gametocytes within the blood. Fertilization and sexual recombination of the parasite occurs in the mosquito's gut. New sporozoites develop and travel to the mosquito's salivary gland, completing the cycle. Pregnant women are especially attractive to the mosquitoes, and malaria in pregnant women is an important cause of stillbirths, infant mortality and low birth weight, particularly in *P. falciparum* infection, but also in other species infection, such as *P. vivax*.

Genetic resistance

Malaria is thought to have been the greatest selective pressure on the human genome in recent history This is due to the high levels of mortality and morbidity caused by malaria, especially the *P. falciparum* species. A number of diseases may provide some resistance to it including sickle cell disease, thalassemia's, glucose-6-phosphate dehydrogenase, Duffy antigens, and possibly others.

Diagnosis

The mainstay of malaria diagnosis has been the microscopic examination of blood Although blood is the sample most frequently used to make a diagnosis, both saliva and urine have been investigated as an alternative, less invasive specimens.

Areas that cannot afford laboratory diagnostic tests often use only a history of subjective fever as an indication to treat for malaria. Using Giemsa-stained blood smears from children in Malawi, one study showed that when clinical predictors (rectal temperature, nailbed pallor, and splenomegaly) were used as treatment indications, rather than using only a history of subjective fevers, a correct diagnosis increased from 2% to 41% of cases, and unnecessary treatment for malaria was significantly decreased.

The most economic, preferred, and reliable diagnosis of malaria is microscopic examination of blood films because each of the four major parasite species has distinguishing characteristics. Two sorts of blood film are traditionally used. Thin films are similar to usual blood films and allow species identification because the parasite's appearance is best preserved in this preparation. Thick films allow the microscopist to screen a larger volume of blood and are about eleven times more sensitive than the thin film, so picking up low levels of infection is easier on the thick film, but the appearance of the parasite is much more distorted and therefore distinguishing between the different species can be much more difficult. With the pros and cons of both thick and thin smears taken into consideration, it is imperative to utilize both smears while attempting to make a definitive diagnosis.

From the thick film, an experienced microscopist can detect parasite levels (or parasitemia) as few as 5 parasites/µBlood. Diagnosis of species can be difficult because the early trophozoites ("ring form") of all four species look identical and it is never possible to diagnose species on the basis of a single ring form; species identification is always based on several trophozoites.

One important thing to note is that *P. malariae* and *P. knowlesi* (which is the most common cause of malaria in South-east Asia) look very similar under the microscope. However, *P.knowlesi* parasitemia increases very fast and causes more severe disease than *P. malariae*, so it is important to identify and treat infections quickly. Therefore, modern methods such as PCR (see "Molecular methods" below) or monoclonal antibody panels that can distinguish between the two should be used in this part of the world.

Antigen tests

For areas where microscopy is not available, or where laboratory staff are not experienced at malaria diagnosis, there are commercial antigen detection tests that require only a drop of blood Immunochromatographic tests (also called: Malaria Rapid Diagnostic Tests, Antigen-Capture Assay or "Dipsticks") have been developed, distributed and field-tested.

These tests use finger-stick or venous blood, the completed test takes a total of 15–20 minutes, and the results are read visually as the presence or absence of colored stripes on the dipstick, so they are suitable for use in the field. The threshold of detection by these rapid diagnostic tests is in the range of 100 parasites/µl of blood (commercial kits can range from about 0.002% to 0.1% parasitemia) compared to 5 by thick film microscopy. One disadvantage is that dipstick tests are qualitative but not quantitative – they can determine if parasites are present in the blood, but not how many.

The first rapid diagnostic tests were using *P. falciparum* glutamate dehydrogenase as antigen. PGluDH was soon replaced by *P.falciparum* lactate dehydrogenase, a 33kDa oxidoreductase. It is the last enzyme of the glycolytic pathway, essential for ATP generation and one of the most abundant enzymes expressed by *P.falciparum*.

PLDH does not persist in the blood but clears about the same time as the parasites following successful treatment. The lack of antigen persistence after treatment makes the pLDH test useful in predicting treatment failure. In this respect, pLDH is similar to pGluDH. Depending on which monoclonal antibodies are used, this type of assay can distinguish between all five different species of human malaria parasites, because of antigenic differences between their pLDH isoenzymes.

Molecular methods

Molecular methods are available in some clinical laboratories and rapid real-time assays (for example, QT-NASBA based on the polymerase chain reaction) are being developed with the hope of being able to deploy them in endemic areas.

PCR (and other molecular methods) is more accurate than microscopy. However, it is expensive, and requires a specialized laboratory. Moreover, levels of parasitemia are not necessarily correlative with the progression of disease, particularly when the parasite is able to adhere to blood vessel walls. Therefore, more sensitive, low-tech diagnosis tools need to be developed in order to detect low levels of parasitemia in the field.

Differential

Fever and septic shock are commonly misdiagnosed as severe malaria in Africa, leading to a failure to treat other life-threatening illnesses. In malaria-endemic areas, parasitemia does not ensure a diagnosis of severe malaria, because parasitemia can be incidental to another concurrent disease. Recent investigations suggest that malarial retinopathy is better (collective sensitivity of 95% and specificity of 90%) than any other clinical or laboratory feature in distinguishing malarial from non-malarial coma. *Anopheles*albuminous mosquito feeding on a human arm. This mosquito is a vector of malaria and mosquito control is a very effective way of reducing the incidence of malaria.

Prevention

Methods used in order to prevent the spread of disease, or to protect individuals in areas where malaria is endemic, include prophylactic drugs, mosquito eradication and the prevention of mosquito bites.

The continued existence of malaria in an area requires a combination of high human population density, high mosquito population density and high rates of transmission from humans to mosquitoes and from mosquitoes to humans. If any of these is lowered sufficiently, the parasite will sooner or later disappear from that area, as happened in North America, Europe and much of Middle East. However, unless the parasite is eliminated from the whole world, it could become re-established if conditions revert to a combination that favors the parasite's reproduction Many countries are seeing an increasing number of imported malaria cases owing to extensive travel and migration.

Medications

Several drugs, most of which are also used for the treatment of malaria, can be taken preventively. Modern drugs used include mefloquine (*Lariat*), doxycycline (available generically), and the combination of atovaquone and proguanil hydrochloride (*Malarone*). Doxycycline and the atovaquone and proguanil combination are the best tolerated with mefloquine associated with higher rates of neurological and psychiatric symptoms. The choice of which drug to use depends on which drugs the parasites in the area are resistant to, as well as side-effects and other considerations. The prophylactic effect does not begin immediately upon starting taking the drugs, so people temporarily visiting malaria-endemic areas usually begin taking the drugs one to two weeks before arriving and must continue taking them for 4 weeks after leaving (with the exception of atovaquone proguanil that only needs be started 2 days prior and continued for 7 days afterwards).

Generally, these drugs are taken daily or weekly, at a lower dose than would be used for treatment of a person who had actually contracted the disease. Use of prophylactic drugs is seldom practical for full-time residents of malaria-endemic areas, and their use is usually restricted to short-term visitors and travelers to malarial regions.

Quinine was used historically, however the development of more effective alternatives such as quinacrine, chloroquine, and primaquine in the 20th century reduced its use.

Indoor residual spraying

Indoor residual spraying (IRS) is the practice of spraying insecticides on the interior walls of homes in malaria affected areas. After feeding, many mosquitos species rest on a nearby surface while digesting the bloodmeal, so if the walls of dwellings have been coated with insecticides, the resting mosquitos will be killed before they can bite another victim, transferring the malaria parasite.

Although DDT has never been banned for use in malaria control and there are several other insecticides suitable for IRS, some advocates have claimed that bans are responsible for tens of millions of deaths in tropical countries where DDT had once been effective in controlling malaria. Furthermore, most of the problems associated with DDT use stem specifically from its industrial-scale application in agriculture, rather than its use in public health.

Mosquito nets and bedclothes

Mosquito nets help keep mosquitoes away from people and greatly reduce the infection and transmission of malaria. The nets are not a perfect barrier and they are often treated with an insecticide designed to kill the mosquito before it has time to search for a way past the net. Insecticide-treated nets (ITNs) are estimated to be twice as effective as untreated nets and offer greater than 70% protection compared with no net. Although ITNs are proven to be very effective against malaria, less than 2% of children in urban areas in Sub-Saharan Africa are protected by ITNs. Since the *Anopheles* mosquitoes feed at night, the preferred method is to hang a large "bed net" above the center of a bed such that it drapes down and covers the bed completely.

Vaccination

Immunity (or, more accurately, tolerance) does occur naturally, but only in response to repeated infection with multiple strains of malaria. Vaccines for malaria are under development, with no completely effective vaccine yet available. It was determined that an individual can be protected from a *P. falciparum* infection if they receive over 1,000 bites from infected yet irradiated mosquitoes.

Other methods

Education in recognizing the symptoms of malaria has reduced the number of cases in some areas of the developing world by as much as 20%. Recognizing the disease in the early stages can also stop the disease from becoming a killer. Education can also inform people to cover over areas of stagnant, still water e.g. Water Tanks which are ideal breeding grounds for the parasite and mosquito, thus cutting down the risk of the transmission between people. This is most put in practice in urban areas where there are large centers of population in a confined space and transmission would be most likely in these areas.

Typhoid fever

Typhoid fever, also known as typhoid is a common worldwide illness, transmitted by the ingestion of food or water contaminated with the feces of an infected person, which contain the bacterium *Salmonella enterica*, serovar Typhi. The bacteria then perforate through the intestinal wall and are phagocytosed by macrophages. The organism is a Gram-negative short bacillus that is motile due to its peritrichous flagella. The bacterium grows best at 37°C / 98.6°F– human body temperature.

This fever received various names, such as gastric fever, abdominal typhus, infantile remittent fever, slow fever, nervous fever, pathogenic fever, etc. The name of "typhoid" comes from the neuropsychiatric symptoms common to typhoid and typhus

The impact of this disease fell sharply with the application of modern sanitation techniques.

Signs and symptoms

Typhoid fever is characterized by a slowly progressive fever as high as 40 °C (104 °F), profuse sweating and gastroenteritis. Less commonly, a rash of flat, rose-colored spots may appear.

Classically, the course of untreated typhoid fever is divided into four individual stages, each lasting approximately one week. In the first week, there is a slowly rising temperature with

relative bradycardia, malaise, headache, and cough. A bloody nose (epistaxis) is seen in a quarter of cases and abdominal pain is also possible. There is leukopenia, a decrease in the number of circulating white blood cells, with eosinopenia and relative lymphocytosis, a positive reaction and blood cultures are positive

for *Salmonella typhi* or *paratyphoid*. The classic Widal test is negative in the first week.

In the second week of the infection, the patient lies prostrate with high fever in plateau around 40

°C (104 °F) and bradycardia (sphygmothermic dissociation), classically with a dicrotic pulse wave. Delirium is frequent, frequently calm, but sometimes agitated. This delirium gives to typhoid the nickname of "nervous fever". Rose spots appear on the lower chest and abdomen in around a third of patients. There are rhonchi in lung bases. The abdomen is distended and painful in the right lower quadrant where borborygmi can be heard. Diarrhea can occur in this stage: six to eight stools in a day, green with a characteristic smell, comparable to pea soup. However, constipation is also frequent. The spleen and liver are enlarged (hepatosplenomegaly) and tender, and there is elevation of liver transaminases. The Widal reaction is strongly positive with antiO and antiH antibodies. Blood cultures are sometimes still positive at this stage. (The major symptom of this fever is that the fever usually rises in the afternoon up to the first and second week.)

In the third week of typhoid fever, a number of complications can occur:

Intestinal hemorrhage due to bleeding in congested Peyer's patches; this can be very serious but is usually not fatal.

Intestinal perforation in the distal ileum: this is a very serious complication and is frequently fatal. It may occur without alarming symptoms until septicemia or diffuse peritonitis sets in.

Encephalitis

Neuropsychiatric symptoms (described as "muttering delirium" or "coma vigil"), with picking at bedclothes or imaginary objects.

Metastatic abscesses, cholecystitis, endocarditis and osteitis

The fever is still very high and oscillates very little over 24 hours. Dehydration ensues and the patient is delirious (typhoid state). By the end of third week the fever has started reducing this. This carries on into the fourth and final week.

Transmission

Flying insects feeding on feces may occasionally transfer the bacteria through poor hygiene habits and public sanitation conditions. Public education campaigns encouraging people to wash their hands after defecating and before handling food are an important component in controlling spread of the disease.

A person may become an asymptomatic carrier of typhoid fever, suffering no symptoms, but capable of infecting others. According to the CDC approximately 5% of people who contract typhoid continue to carry the disease after they recover. The most famous asymptomatic carrier was Mary Mallon (commonly known as "Typhoid Mary"), a young cook who was responsible for infecting at least 53 people with typhoid, three of whom died from the disease. Mallon was the first apparently perfectly healthy person known to be responsible for an "epidemic".

Many carriers of typhoid were locked into an isolation ward never to be released in order to prevent further typhoid cases. These people often deteriorated mentally, driven mad by the conditions they lived in.

Possible protective effects of heterozygosity for cystic fibrosis

It has been hypothesized that cystic fibrosis may have risen to its present levels due to the heterozygous advantage that it confers against typhoid fever. The CFTR protein is present in both the lungs and the intestinal epithelium, and the mutant cystic fibrosis form of the CFTR protein prevents entry of the typhoid bacterium into the body through the intestinal epithelium. However, the heterozygous advantage hypothesis was proposed in one review in which the author himself writes, "Although cellular/molecular evidence presented is not available for this hypothesis, the CF mutation may be one of several mutations that have spread in European populations because they increased resistance to infectious diseases." Since no molecular experimental evidence has been presented in support of this theory; this theory is not accepted by the majority of the scientific community.

Diagnosis of typhoid

Diagnosis is made by any blood, bone marrow or stool cultures and with the Widal test (demonstration of salmonella antibodies against antigens O-somatic and H-flagellar). In epidemics and less wealthy countries, after excluding malaria, dysentery or pneumonia, a therapeutic trial time with chloramphenicol is generally undertaken while awaiting the results of the Widal test and cultures of the blood and stool.

The Widal test is time-consuming and oftentimes when diagnosis is reached it is too late to start an antibiotic regimen.

The term "enteric fever" is a collective term that refers to typhoid and paratyphoid.

Prevention

Sanitation and hygiene are the critical measures that can be taken to prevent typhoid. Typhoid does not affect animals and therefore transmission is only from human to human. Typhoid can only spread in environments where human feces or urine are able to come into contact with food or drinking water. Careful food preparation and washing of hands are crucial to preventing typhoid.

There are two vaccines currently recommended by the World Health Organization for the prevention of typhoid: these are the live, oral Ty21a vaccine (sold as *Vivotif Berna*) and the injectable Typhoid polysaccharide vaccine (sold as *Typhi Vi* by Sanofi Pasteur and *Typherix* by GlaxoSmithKline). Both are between 50% to 80% protective and are recommended for travelers to areas where typhoid is endemic.

Boosters are recommended every 5 years for the oral vaccine and every 2 years for the injectable form. There exists an older killed whole-cell vaccine that is still used in countries where the newer preparations are not available, but this vaccine is no longer recommended for use, because it has a higher rate of side effects (mainly pain and inflammation at the site of the injection).

Treatment

The rediscovery of oral rehydration therapy in the 1960s provided a simple way to prevent many of the deaths of diarrheal diseases in general.

Where resistance is uncommon, the treatment of choice is a fluoroquinolone such as ciprofloxacin otherwise, a third-generation cephalosporin such as ceftriaxone or cefotaxime is the first choice Cefixime is a suitable oral alternative Typhoid fever in most cases is not fatal. Antibiotics, such as ampicillin, chloramphenicol, trimethoprim-sulfamethoxazole, Amoxicillin and ciprofloxacin, have been commonly used to treat typhoid fever in developed countries. Prompt treatment of the disease with antibiotics reduces the case-fatality rate to approximately 1%.

When untreated, typhoid fever persists for three weeks to a month. Death occurs in between 10% and 30% of untreated cases[In some communities, however, case-fatality rates may reach as high as 47%.

Resistance

Resistance to ampicillin, chloramphenicol, trimethoprim-sulfamethoxazole and streptomycin is now common, and these agents have not been used as first line treatment now for almost 20 years Typhoid that is resistant to these agents is known as multidrug-resistant typhoid (MDR typhoid).

Ciprofloxacin resistance is an increasing problem, especially in the Indian subcontinent and Southeast Asia. Many centers are therefore moving away from using ciprofloxacin as first line for treating suspected typhoid originating in South America, India, Pakistan, Bangladesh, Thailand or Vietnam. For these patients, the recommended first line treatment is ceftriaxone. It has also been suggested Azithromycin is better at treating typhoid in resistant populations than both fluoroquinolone drugs and ceftriaxone.[18]Azithromycin significantly reduces relapse rates compared with ceftriaxone.

There is a separate problem with laboratory testing for reduced susceptibility to ciprofloxacin: current recommendations are that isolates should be tested simultaneously against ciprofloxacin (CIP) and against nalidixic acid (NAL), and that isolates that are sensitive to both CIP and NAL should be reported as "sensitive to ciprofloxacin", but that isolates testing sensitive to CIP but not to NAL should be reported as

"reduced sensitivity to ciprofloxacin". However, an analysis of 271 isolates showed that around 18% of isolates with reduced susceptibility to ciprofloxacin (MIC 0.125–1.0 mg/l) would not be picked up by this method. It is not certain how this problem can be solved because most laboratories around the world (including the West) are dependent on disc testing and cannot test for MICs.

CHAPTER TWELVE

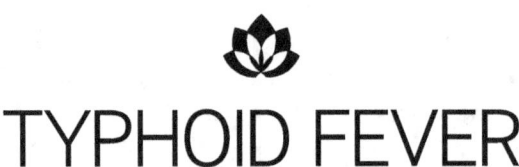

TYPHOID FEVER

Typhoid fever

Typhoid fever, also known as typhoid is a common worldwide illness, transmitted by the ingestion of food or water contaminated with the feces of an infected person, which contain the bacterium *Salmonella enterica*, serovar Typhi. The bacteria then perforate through the intestinal wall and are phagocytosed by macrophages. The organism is a Gram-negative short bacillus that is motile due to its peritrichous flagella. The bacterium grows best at 37°C / 98.6°F– human body temperature.

This fever received various names, such as gastric fever, abdominal typhus, infantile remittent fever, slow fever, nervous fever, pathogenic fever, etc. The name of "typhoid" comes from the neuropsychiatric symptoms common to typhoid and typhus

The impact of this disease fell sharply with the application of modern sanitation techniques.

Signs and symptoms

Typhoid fever is characterized by a slowly progressive fever as high as 40 °C (104 °F), profuse sweating and gastroenteritis. Less commonly, a rash of flat, rose-colored spots may appear.

Classically, the course of untreated typhoid fever is divided into four individual stages, each lasting approximately one week. In the first week, there is a slowly rising temperature with

relative bradycardia, malaise, headache, and cough. A bloody nose (epistaxis) is seen in a quarter of cases and abdominal pain is also possible. There is leukopenia, a decrease in the number of circulating white blood cells, with eosinopenia and relative lymphocytosis, a positive reaction and blood cultures are positive

for *Salmonella typhi* or *paratyphoid*. The classic Widal test is negative in the first week.

In the second week of the infection, the patient lies prostrate with high fever in plateau around 40 °C (104 °F) and bradycardia (sphygmothermic dissociation), classically with a dicrotic pulse wave. Delirium is frequent, frequently calm, but sometimes agitated. This delirium gives to typhoid the nickname of "nervous fever". Rose spots appear on the lower chest and abdomen in around a third of patients. There are rhonchi in lung bases. The abdomen is distended and painful in the right lower quadrant where borborygmi can be heard. Diarrhea can occur in this stage: six to eight stools in a day, green with a characteristic smell, comparable to pea soup. However, constipation is also frequent. The spleen and liver are enlarged (hepatosplenomegaly) and tender, and there is elevation of liver transaminases. The Widal reaction is strongly positive with antiO and antiH antibodies. Blood cultures are sometimes still positive at this stage. (The major symptom of this fever is that the fever usually rises in the afternoon up to the first and second week.)

In the third week of typhoid fever, a number of complications can occur:

    Intestinal hemorrhage due to bleeding in congested Peyer's patches; this can be very serious but is usually not fatal.

    Intestinal perforation in the distal ileum: this is a very serious complication and is frequently fatal. It may occur without alarming symptoms until septicemia or diffuse peritonitis sets in.

    Encephalitis

Neuropsychiatric symptoms (described as "muttering delirium" or "coma vigil"), with picking at bedclothes or imaginary objects.

Metastatic abscesses, cholecystitis, endocarditis and osteitis

The fever is still very high and oscillates very little over 24 hours. Dehydration ensues and the patient is delirious (typhoid state). By the end of third week the fever has started reducing this. This carries on into the fourth and final week.

Transmission

Flying insects feeding on feces may occasionally transfer the bacteria through poor hygiene habits and public sanitation conditions. Public education campaigns encouraging people to wash their hands after defecating and before handling food are an important component in controlling spread of the disease.

A person may become an asymptomatic carrier of typhoid fever, suffering no symptoms, but capable of infecting others. According to the CDC approximately 5% of people who contract typhoid continue to carry the disease after they recover. The most famous asymptomatic carrier was Mary Mallon (commonly known as "Typhoid Mary"), a young cook who was responsible for infecting at least 53 people with typhoid, three of whom died from the disease. Mallon was the first apparently perfectly healthy person known to be responsible for an "epidemic".

Many carriers of typhoid were locked into an isolation ward never to be released in order to prevent further typhoid cases. These people often deteriorated mentally, driven mad by the conditions they lived in.

Possible protective effects of heterozygosity for cystic fibrosis

It has been hypothesized that cystic fibrosis may have risen to its present levels due to the heterozygous advantage that it confers against typhoid fever. The CFTR protein is present in both the lungs and the intestinal epithelium, and the mutant cystic fibrosis form of the CFTR protein prevents entry of the typhoid bacterium into the body through the intestinal epithelium. However, the heterozygous advantage hypothesis was proposed in one review in which the author himself writes, "Although cellular/molecular evidence presented is not available for this hypothesis, the CF mutation may be one of several mutations that have spread in European populations because they increased resistance to infectious diseases." Since no molecular experimental evidence has been presented in support of this theory; this theory is not accepted by the majority of the scientific community.

Diagnosis of typhoid

Diagnosis is made by any blood, bone marrow or stool cultures and with the Widal test (demonstration of salmonella antibodies against antigens O-somatic and H-flagellar). In epidemics and less wealthy countries, after excluding malaria, dysentery or pneumonia, a therapeutic trial time with chloramphenicol is generally undertaken while awaiting the results of the Widal test and cultures of the blood and stool.

The Widal test is time-consuming and oftentimes when diagnosis is reached it is too late to start an antibiotic regimen.

The term "enteric fever" is a collective term that refers to typhoid and paratyphoid.

Prevention

Sanitation and hygiene are the critical measures that can be taken to prevent typhoid. Typhoid does not affect animals and therefore transmission is only from human to human. Typhoid can only spread in environments where human feces or urine are able to come into contact with food or drinking water. Careful food preparation and washing of hands are crucial to preventing typhoid.

There are two vaccines currently recommended by the World Health Organization for the prevention of typhoid: these are the live, oral Ty21a vaccine (sold as *Vivotif Berna*) and the injectable Typhoid polysaccharide vaccine (sold as *Typhi Vi* by Sanofi Pasteur and *Typherix* by GlaxoSmithKline). Both are between 50% to 80% protective and are recommended for travelers to areas where typhoid is endemic.

Boosters are recommended every 5 years for the oral vaccine and every 2 years for the injectable form. There exists an older killed whole-cell vaccine that is still used in countries where the newer preparations are not available, but this vaccine is no longer recommended for use, because it has a higher rate of side effects (mainly pain and inflammation at the site of the injection).

Treatment

The rediscovery of oral rehydration therapy in the 1960s provided a simple way to prevent many of the deaths of diarrheal diseases in general.

Where resistance is uncommon, the treatment of choice is a fluoroquinolone such as ciprofloxacin otherwise, a third-generation cephalosporin such as ceftriaxone or cefotaxime is the first choice Cefixime is a suitable oral alternative Typhoid fever in most cases is not fatal. Antibiotics, such as ampicillin, chloramphenicol, trimethoprim-sulfamethoxazole, Amoxicillin and ciprofloxacin, have been commonly used to treat typhoid fever in developed countries. Prompt treatment of the disease with antibiotics reduces the case-fatality rate to approximately 1%.

When untreated, typhoid fever persists for three weeks to a month. Death occurs in between 10% and 30% of untreated cases[In some communities, however, case-fatality rates may reach as high as 47%.

Resistance

Resistance to ampicillin, chloramphenicol, trimethoprim-sulfamethoxazole and streptomycin is now common, and these agents have not been used as first line treatment now for almost 20 years Typhoid that is resistant to these agents is known as multidrug-resistant typhoid (MDR typhoid).

Ciprofloxacin resistance is an increasing problem, especially in the Indian subcontinent and Southeast Asia. Many centers are therefore moving away from using ciprofloxacin as first line for treating suspected typhoid originating in South America, India, Pakistan, Bangladesh, Thailand or Vietnam. For these patients, the recommended first line treatment is ceftriaxone. It has also been suggested Azithromycin is better at treating typhoid in resistant populations than both fluoroquinolone drugs and ceftriaxone.[18]Azithromycin significantly reduces relapse rates compared with ceftriaxone.

There is a separate problem with laboratory testing for reduced susceptibility to ciprofloxacin: current recommendations are that isolates should be tested simultaneously against ciprofloxacin (CIP) and against nalidixic acid (NAL), and that isolates that are sensitive to both CIP and NAL should be reported as "sensitive to ciprofloxacin", but that isolates testing sensitive to CIP but not to NAL should be reported as

"reduced sensitivity to ciprofloxacin". However, an analysis of 271 isolates showed that around 18% of isolates with reduced susceptibility to ciprofloxacin (MIC 0.125–1.0 mg/l) would not be picked up by this method. It is not certain how this problem can be solved because most laboratories around the world (including the West) are dependent on disc testing and cannot test for MICs.

CHAPTER THIRTEEN

Acquired immunodeficiency syndrome (AIDS)

Acquired immune deficiency syndrome or acquired immunodeficiency syndrome (AIDS) is a disease of the human immune system caused by the human immunodeficiency virus (HIV This condition progressively reduces the effectiveness of the immune system and leaves individuals susceptible to opportunistic infections and tumours. HIV is transmitted through direct contact of a mucous membrane or the bloodstream with a bodily fluid containing HIV, such as blood, semen, vaginal fluid, pre-seminal fluid, and breast milk. This transmission can involve anal, vaginal or oral sex, blood transfusion, contaminated hypodermic needles, exchange between mother and baby during pregnancy, childbirth, breastfeeding or other exposure to one of the above bodily fluids.

Although treatments for AIDS and HIV can slow the course of the disease, there is no known cure or vaccine. Antiretroviral treatment reduces both the mortality and the morbidity of HIV infection, but these drugs are expensive and routine access to antiretroviral medication is not available in all countries. Due to the difficulty in treating HIV infection, preventing infection is a key aim in controlling the AIDS pandemic, with health organizations promoting safe sex and needle-exchange programmes in attempts to slow the spread of the virus.

Main symptoms of AIDS

The symptoms of AIDS are primarily the result of conditions that do not normally develop in individuals with healthy immune systems. Most of these conditions are infections caused by bacteria, viruses, fungi and parasites that are normally controlled by the elements of the immune system that HIV damages.

Opportunistic infections are common in people with AIDS. These infections affect nearly every organ system.

People with AIDS also have an increased risk of developing various cancers such as Kaposi's sarcoma, cervical cancer and cancers of the immune system known as lymphomas. Additionally, people with AIDS often have systemic symptoms of infection like fevers, sweats (particularly at night), swollen glands, chills, weakness, and weight loss. The specific opportunistic infections that AIDS patients develop depend in part on the prevalence of these infections in the geographic area in which the patient lives.

Pulmonary

Pneumocystis pneumonia (originally known as *Pneumocystis carinii* pneumonia, and still abbreviated as PCP, which now stands for Pneumocystis pneumonia) is relatively rare in healthy, immunocompetent people, but common among HIV-infected individuals. It is caused by *Pneumocystis jirovecii*.

Before the advent of effective diagnosis, treatment and routine prophylaxis in Western countries, it was a common immediate cause of death. In developing countries, it is still one of the first indications of AIDS in untested individuals, although it does not generally occur unless the CD4 count is less than 200 cells per μL of blood.

Tuberculosis (TB) is unique among infections associated with HIV because it is transmissible to immunocompetent people via the respiratory route, and is not easily treatable once identified,[45]Multidrug resistance is a serious problem. Tuberculosis with HIV co-infection (TB/HIV) is a major world health problem according to the World Health Organization: in 2007, 456,000 deaths among incident TB cases were HIV-positive, a third of all TB deaths and nearly a quarter of the estimated 2 million HIV deaths in that year

Even though its incidence has declined because of the use of directly observed therapy and other improved practices in Western countries, this is not the case in developing countries where HIV is most prevalent. In early-stage HIV infection (CD4 count >300 cells per µL), TB typically presents as a pulmonary disease. In advanced HIV infection, TB often presents atypically with extrapulmonary (systemic) disease a common feature. Symptoms are usually constitutional and are not localized to one particular site, often affecting bone marrow, bone, urinary and gastrointestinal tracts, liver, regional lymph nodes, and the central nervous system

Gastrointestinal

Esophagitis is an inflammation of the lining of the lower end of the esophagus (gullet or swallowing tube leading to the stomach). In HIV-infected individuals, this is normally due to fungal (candidiasis) or viral (herpes simplex-1 or cytomegalovirus) infections. In rare cases, it could be due to mycobacteria.

Unexplained chronic diarrhea in HIV infection is due to many possible causes, including common bacterial (*Salmonella, Shigella, Listeria* or*Campylobacter*) and parasitic infections; and uncommon opportunistic infections such as cryptosporidiosis, microsporidiosis, *Mycobacterium avium* complex (MAC) and viruses, astrovirus, adenovirus, rotavirus and cytomegalovirus, (the latter as a course of colitis).

In some cases, diarrhea may be a side effect of several drugs used to treat HIV, or it may simply accompany HIV infection, particularly during primary HIV infection. It may also be a side effect of antibiotics used to treat bacterial causes of diarrhea (common for *Clostridium difficile*). In the later stages of HIV infection, diarrhea is thought to be a reflection of changes in the way

the intestinal tract absorbs nutrients, and may be an important component of HIV-related wasting.

Neurological and psychiatric

HIV infection may lead to a variety of neuropsychiatric sequelae, either by infection of the now susceptible nervous system by organisms, or as a direct consequence of the illness itself

To

AIDS dementia complex (ADC) is a metabolic encephalopathy induced by HIV infection and fueled by immune activation of HIV infected brain macrophages and microglia. These cells are productively infected by HIV and secrete neurotoxins of both host and viral origin. Specific neurological impairments are manifested by cognitive, behavioral, and motor abnormalities that occur after years of HIV infection and are associated with low $CD4^+T$ cell levels and high plasma viral loads.

Prevalence is 10–20% in Western countries but only 1–2% of HIV infections in India. This difference is possibly due to the HIV subtype in India. AIDS-related mania is sometimes seen in patients with advanced HIV illness; it presents with more irritability and cognitive impairment and less euphoria than a manic episode associated with true bipolar disorder. Unlike the latter condition, it may have a more chronic course. This syndrome is less often seen with the advent of multi-drug therapy.

Tumors in Aids

Patients with HIV infection have substantially increased incidence of several cancers. This is primarily due to co-infection with an oncogenic DNA virus, especially Epstein-Barr virus (EBV), Kaposi's sarcoma-associated herpesvirus (KSHV) (also known as human herpesvirus-8 [HHV-8]), and human papillomavirus (HPV).

Kaposi's sarcoma (KS) is the most common tumor in HIV-infected patients. The appearance of this tumor in young homosexual men in 1981 was one of the first signals of the AIDS epidemic. Caused by a gamma herpes virus called Kaposi's sarcoma- associated herpes virus (KSHV), it often appears as purplish nodules on the skin, but can affect other organs, especially the mouth, gastrointestinal tract, and lungs. High-grade B cell lymphomas such as Burkitt's lymphoma, Burkitt's-like lymphoma, diffuse large B-cell lymphoma (DLBCL), and primary central nervous system lymphoma present more often in HIV-infected patients. These particular cancers often foreshadow a poor prognosis. Epstein-Barr virus (EBV) or KSHV cause many of these lymphomas. In HIV-infected patients, lymphoma often arises in extranidal sites such as the gastrointestinal tract. When they occur in an HIV-infected patient, KS and aggressive B cell lymphomas confer a diagnosis of AIDS.

Invasive cervical cancer in HIV-infected women is also considered AIDS-defining, it is caused by human papillomavirus (HPV).

Other infections

AIDS patients often develop opportunistic infections that present with non-specific symptoms, especially low-grade fevers and weight loss. These include opportunistic infection with *Mycobacterium avium-intracellular* and cytomegalovirus (CMV). CMV can cause colitis, as described above, and CMV retinitis can cause blindness.

Penicilloic due to *Penicillium Menefee* is now the third most common opportunistic infection (after extrapulmonary tuberculosis and cryptococcosis) in HIV-positive individuals within the endemic area of Southeast Asia. An infection that often goes unrecognized in AIDS patients is Parvovirus B19. Its main consequence is anemia, which is difficult to distinguish from the effects of antiretroviral drugs used to treat AIDS itself.

Cause

A generalized graph of the relationship between HIV copies (viral load) and CD4 counts over the average course of untreated HIV infection; any particular individual's disease course may vary considerably. $CD4^+T$ Lymphocyte count (cells/mm³) HIV RNA copies per mL of plasma

AIDS is the ultimate clinical consequence of infection with HIV. HIV is a retrovirus that primarily infects vital organs of the human immune system such as $CD4^+T$ cells (a subset of T cells), macrophages and dendritic cells. It directly and indirectly destroys $CD4^+T$ cells

Once the number of $CD4^+T$ cells per microliter (μL) of blood drops below 200, cellular immunity is lost. Acute HIV infection usually progresses over time to clinical latent HIV infection and then to early symptomatic HIV infection and later to AIDS, which is identified either on the basis of the amount of $CD4^+T$ cells remaining in the blood, and/or the presence of certain infections, as noted above

In the absence of antiretroviral therapy, the median time of progression from HIV infection to AIDSs nine to ten years, and the median survival time after developing AIDS is only 9.2 months. However, the rate of clinical disease progression varies widely between individuals, from two weeks up to 20 years.

Many factors affect the rate of progression. These include factors that influence the body's ability to defend against HIV such as the infected person's general immune function. Older people have weaker immune systems, and therefore have a greater risk of rapid disease progression than younger people.

Poor access to health care and the existence of coexisting infections such as tuberculosis also may predispose people to faster disease progression. The infected person's genetic inheritance plays an important role and some people are resistant to certain strains of HIV. An example of this is people with the homozygous CCR5-Δ32 variation are resistant to infection with certain strains of HIV.[72] HIV is genetically variable and exists as different strains, which cause different rates of clinical disease progression.

There are a number HIV and AIDS misconceptions. Three of the most common are that AIDS can spread through casual contact, that sexual intercourse with a virgin will cure AIDS, and that HIV can infect only homosexual men and drug users. Other misconceptions are that any act of anal intercourse between gay men can lead to AIDS infection, and that open discussion of homosexuality and HIV in schools will lead to increased rates of homosexuality and AIDS.

sexual transmission

Sexual transmission occurs with the contact between sexual secretions of one person with the rectal, genital or oral mucous membranes of another. Unprotected sexual acts are riskier for the receptive partner than for the insertive partner, and the risk for transmitting HIV through unprotected anal intercourse is greater than the risk from vaginal intercourse or oral sex. However, oral sex is not entirely safe, as HIV can be transmitted through both insertive and receptive oral sex

Sexual assault greatly increases the risk of HIV transmission as condoms are rarely employed and physical trauma to the vagina or rectum occurs frequently, facilitating the transmission of HIV.

Drug use has been studied as a possible predictor of HIV transmission. Perry N. Halkitis found that methamphetamine usage does significantly relate to unprotected sexual behavior. The study found methamphetamine users to be at a higher risk for contracting HIV.

Other sexually transmitted infections (STI) increase the risk of HIV transmission and infection, because they cause the disruption of the normal epithelial barrier by genital ulceration and/or microulceration; and by accumulation of pools of HIV-susceptible or HIV-infected cells (lymphocytes and macrophages) in semen and vaginal secretions. Epidemiological studies from sub-Saharan

Africa, Europe and North America suggest that genital ulcers, such as those caused by syphilis and/or chancroid, increase the risk of becoming infected with HIV by about fourfold. There is also a significant although lesser increase in risk from STIs such as gonorrhea, chlamydia and trichomoniasis, which all cause local accumulations of lymphocytes and macrophages.

Transmission of HIV depends on the infectiousness of the index case and the susceptibility of the uninfected partner. Infectivity seems to vary during the course of illness and is not constant between individuals. An undetectable plasma viral load does not necessarily indicate a low viral load in the seminal liquid or genital secretions.

Infection is unlikely in a single encounter. High rates of infection have been linked to a pattern of overlapping long-term sexual relationships. This allows the virus to quickly spread to multiple partners who in turn infect their partners. A pattern of serial monogamy or occasional casual encounters is associated with lower rates of infection.

HIV spreads readily through heterosexual sex in Africa, but less so elsewhere. One possibility being researched is that schistosomiasis, which affects up to 50% of women in parts of Africa, damages the lining of the vagina.

Blood products

This transmission route is particularly relevant to intravenous drug users, haemophiliacs and recipients of blood transfusions and blood products. Sharing and reusing syringes contaminated with HIV-infected blood represents a major risk for infection with HIV.

Perinatal transmission

The transmission of the virus from the mother to the child can occur *in utero* during the last weeks of pregnancy and at childbirth. In the absence of treatment, the transmission rate between a mother and her child during pregnancy, labor and delivery is 25%. However, when the mother takes antiretroviral therapy and gives birth by caesarean section, the rate of transmission is just 1%.

The risk of infection is influenced by the viral load of the mother at birth, with the higher the viral load, the higher the risk. Breastfeeding also increases the risk of transmission by about 4 %.

Pathophysiology

The pathophysiology of AIDS is complex, as is the case with all syndromes. Ultimately, HIV causes AIDS by depleting $CD4^+T$ helper lymphocytes. This weakens the immune system and allows opportunistic infections. T lymphocytes are essential to the immune response and without them, the body cannot fight infections or kill cancerous cells. The mechanism of $CD4^+T$ cell depletion differs in the acute and chronic phases.

During the acute phase, HIV-induced cell lysis and killing of infected cells by cytotoxic T cells accounts for $CD4^+T$ cell depletion, although apoptosis may also be a factor. During the chronic phase, the consequences of generalized immune activation coupled with the gradual loss of the ability of the immune system to generate new T cells appear to account for the slow decline in CD4⁺T cell numbers.

Although the symptoms of immune deficiency characteristic of AIDS do not appear for years after a person is infected, the bulk of CD4⁺T cell loss occurs during the first weeks of infection, especially in the intestinal mucosa, which harbors the majority of the lymphocytes found in the body The reason for the preferential loss of mucosal CD4⁺T cells is that a majority of mucosal CD4⁺T cells express the CCR5 coreceptor, whereas a small fraction of CD4⁺T cells in the bloodstream do so.

HIV seeks out and destroys CCR5 expressing CD4⁺cells during acute infection. A vigorous immune response eventually controls the infection and initiates the clinically latent phase. However, CD4⁺T cells in mucosal tissues remain depleted throughout the infection, although enough remain to initially ward off life-threatening infections.

Continuous HIV replication results in a state of generalized immune activation persisting throughout the chronic phase. Immune activation, which is reflected by the increased activation state of immune cells and release of proinflammatory cytokines, results from the activity of several HIV gene products and the immune response to ongoing HIV replication. Another cause is the breakdown of the immune surveillance system of the mucosal barrier caused by the depletion of mucosal CD4⁺T cells during the acute phase of disease

Diagnosis

The diagnosis of AIDS in a person infected with HIV is based on the presence of certain signs or symptoms. Since June 5, 1981, many definitions have been developed for epidemiological surveillance such as the Bangui definition and the 1994 expanded World

Health Organization AIDS case definition. However, clinical staging of patients was not an intended use for these systems as they are neither sensitive, nor specific. In developing countries, the World Health Organization staging system for HIV infection and disease, using clinical and laboratory data, is used and in developed countries, the Centers for Disease Control (CDC) Classification System is used.

HIV test

Many people are unaware that they are infected with HIV. Less than 1% of the sexually active urban population in Africa has been tested, and this proportion is even lower in rural populations. Furthermore, only 0.5% of pregnant women attending urban health facilities are counseled, tested or receive their test results. Again, this proportion is even lower in rural health facilities. Therefore, donor blood and blood products used in medicine and medical research are screened for HIV.

HIV tests are usually performed on venous blood. Many laboratories use *fourth generation* screening tests which detect anti-HIV antibody (IgG and IgM) and the HIV p24 antigen. The detection of HIV antibody or antigen in a patient previously known to be negative is evidence of HIV infection. Individuals whose first specimen indicates evidence of HIV infection will have a repeat test on a second blood sample to confirm the results.

The window period (the time between initial infection and the development of detectable antibodies against the infection) can vary since it can take 3–6 months to seroconvert and to test positive. Detection of the virus using polymerase chain reaction (PCR) during the window period is possible, and evidence suggests that an infection may often be detected earlier than when using a fourth generation EIA screening test.

Positive results obtained by PCR are confirmed by antibody tests. Routinely used HIV tests for infection in neonates and infants (i.e., patients younger than 2 years born to HIV-positive mothers, have no value because of the presence of maternal antibody to HIV in the child's blood. HIV infection can only be diagnosed by PCR, testing for HIV pro-viral DNA in the children's lymphocytes.

Prevention

The three main transmission routes of HIV are sexual contact, exposure to infected body fluids or tissues, and from mother to fetus or child during perinatal period. It is possible to find HIV in the saliva, tears, and urine of infected individuals, but there are no recorded cases of infection by these secretions, and the risk of infection is negligible. Anti-retroviral treatment of infected patients also significantly reduces their ability to transmit HIV to others, by reducing the amount of virus in their bodily fluids to undetectable levels.

Sexual contact

The majority of HIV infections are acquired through unprotected sexual relations between partners, one of whom has HIV. The primary mode of HIV infection worldwide is through sexual contact between members of the opposite sex.

During a sexual act, only male or female condoms can reduce the risk of infection with HIV and other STDs. The best evidence to date indicates that typical condom use reduces the risk of heterosexual HIV transmission by approximately 80% over the long-term, though the benefit is likely to be higher if condoms are used correctly on every occasion.

The male latex condom, if used correctly without oil-based lubricants, is the single most effective available technology to reduce the sexual transmission of HIV and other sexually transmitted infections. Manufacturers recommend that oil-based lubricants such as petroleum jelly, butter, and lard not be used with latex condoms, because they dissolve the latex, making the condoms porous. If lubrication is desired, manufacturers recommend using water-based lubricants. Oil-based lubricants can be used with polyurethane condoms.

Female condoms are commonly made from polyurethane, but are also made from nitrile and latex. They are larger than male condoms and have a stiffened ring-shaped opening with an inner ring designed to be inserted into the vagina keeping the condom in place; inserting the female condom requires squeezing this ring. Female condoms have been shown to be an important HIV prevention strategy by preliminary studies which suggest that overall protected sexual acts increase relative to unprotected sexual acts where female condoms are available. At present, availability of female condoms is very low and the price remains prohibitive for many women.

Education

One way to change risky behavior is health education.

Management

There is currently no publicly available vaccine for HIV or cure for HIV or AIDS. The only known methods of prevention are based on avoiding exposure to the virus or, failing that, an antiretroviral treatment directly after a highly significant exposure, called post-exposure prophylaxis (PEP). PEP has a very demanding four-week schedule of dosage. It also has very unpleasant side effects including diarrhea, malaise, nausea and fatigue.

Antiviral therapy

Current treatment for HIV infection consists of highly active antiretroviral therapy, or HAART. This has been highly beneficial to many HIV-infected individuals since its introduction in 1996 when the protease inhibitor-based HAART initially became available. Current optimal HAART options consist of combinations (or "cocktails") consisting of at least three drugs belonging to at least two types, or "classes," of antiretroviral agents.

AIDS stigma exists around the world in a variety of ways, including ostracism, rejection, discrimination and avoidance of HIV infected people; compulsory HIV testing without prior consent or protection of confidentiality; violence against HIV infected individuals or people who are perceived to be infected with HIV; and the quarantine of HIV infected individuals. Stigma-related violence or the fear of violence prevents many people from seeking HIV testing, returning for their results, or securing treatment, possibly turning what could be a manageable chronic illness into a death sentence and perpetuating the spread of HIV. AIDS stigma has been further divided into the following three categories:

Instrumental AIDS stigma—a reflection of the fear and apprehension that are likely to be associated with any deadly and transmissible illness. *Symbolic AIDS stigma*—the use of HIV/AIDS to express attitudes toward the social groups or lifestyles perceived to be associated with the disease. *Courtesy AIDS stigma*—stigmatization of people connected to the issue of HIV/AIDS or HIV-positive people.

CHAPTER FOURTEEN

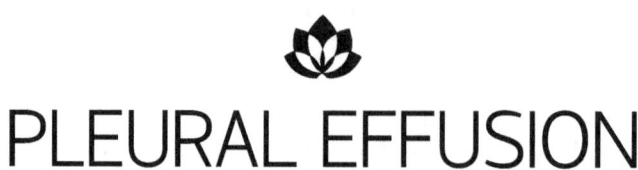

PLEURAL EFFUSION

Pleural effusion is excess fluid that accumulates in the pleura, the fluid-filled space that surrounds the lungs. Excessive amounts of such fluid can impair breathing by limiting the expansion of the lungs during respiration.

Types of fluids
Four types of fluids can accumulate in the pleural space:
Serous fluid (hydrothorax)
Blood (hemothorax)
Chyle (chylothorax)
Pus (pyothorax or empyema)

Diagnosis
Pleural effusion is usually diagnosed on the basis of medical history and physical exam, and confirmed
by chest x-ray. Once accumulated fluid is more than 500 ml, there are usually detectable clinical signs in the patient, such as decreased movement of the chest on the affected side, stony dullness to percussion over the fluid, diminished breath sounds on the affected side, decreased vocal resonance and fremitus(though this is an inconsistent and unreliable sign), and pleural friction rub. Above the effusion, where the lung is compressed,
there may be bronchial breathing and egophony. In large effusion there may be tracheal deviation away from the effusion.
Imaging
Normally the space between the two layers of the lung, the visceral pleura and the parietal pleura, cannot be seen. A pleural effusion infiltrates the space between these layers. Because the pleural effusion has a density similar to body fluid or water, it can be seen on radiographs. Since the effusion has greater density than the rest of the lung, it will gravitate towards the lower portions of the pleural cavity. The pleural effusion behaves according to basic fluid dynamics, conforming to the shape of the lung and chest cavity. If the pleural cavity contains both air and fluid, then the fluid will have a "fluid level" that is horizontal instead of conforming to the lung space. Chest radiographs acquired in the lateral decubitus position (with the patient lying on his side) are more sensitive and can pick up as little as 50 ml of fluid. At least 300 ml of fluid must be present before upright chest films can pick up signs of pleural effusion (e.g., blunted costophrenic angles).
Massive left-sided pleural effusion (whiteness) in a patient presenting with lung cancer.
Thoracentesis
Once a pleural effusion is diagnosed, the cause must be determined. Pleural fluid is drawn out of the pleural space in a process called thoracentesis. A needle is inserted through the back of the chest wall in the sixth, seventh, or eighth intercostal space on the midaxillary line, into the pleural space. The fluid may then be evaluated for the following:
Chemical composition including protein, lactate dehydrogenase (LDH), albumin, amylase, pH, and glucose
Gram stain and culture to identify possible bacterial infections
Cell count and differential
Cytopathology to identify cancer cells, but may also identify some infective organisms

Other tests as suggested by the clinical situation – lipids, fungal culture, viral culture, specific immunoglobulins

Definitions of the terms "transudate" and "exudate" are the source of much confusion. Briefly, transudate is produced through pressure filtration without capillary injury while exudate is "inflammatory fluid" leaking between cells.

Transudative pleural effusions are defined as effusions that are caused by *systemic* factors that alter the pleural equilibrium, or Starling forces. The components of the Starling forces–hydrostatic pressure, permeability, oncotic pressure (effective pressure due to the composition of the pleural fluid and blood)–are altered in many diseases, e.g., left ventricular failure, renal failure, hepatic failure, and cirrhosis. Exudative pleural effusions, by contrast, are caused by alterations in *local* factors that influence the formation and absorption of pleural fluid (e.g., bacterial pneumonia, cancer, pulmonary embolism, and viral infection

Although Light's criteria are relatively accurate, twenty-five percent of patients with transudative pleural effusions are mistakenly identified by Light's criteria as having exudative pleural effusions. Therefore, if a patient identified by Light's criteria as having an exudative pleural effusion appears clinically to have a condition that usually produces transudative effusions, additional testing is needed. In such cases albumin levels in blood and pleural fluid are measured. If the difference between the albumin level in the blood and the pleural fluid is greater than 1.2 g/dL (12 g/L), this suggests that the patient has a transudative pleural effusion. However, pleural fluid testing is not perfect, and the final decision about whether a fluid is a transudate or an exudate is based not on chemical analysis of the fluid, but on accurate diagnosis of the disease that produces the fluid.

Causes
  Transudative
  The most common causes of transudative pleural effusions in the United States are left ventricular failure, and cirrhosis (causing hepatic hydrothorax), nephrotic syndrome leading to increased loss of albumin and resultant hypoalbuminemia and thus reducing colloid osmotic pressure is another less common cause.
  Pulmonary embolisms were once thought to be transudative but have been recently shown to be exudative
  Exudative
  Once identified as exudative, additional evaluation is needed to determine the cause of the excess fluid, and pleural fluid amylase, glucose, pH and cell counts are obtained.
  Pleural fluid amylase is elevated in cases of esophageal rupture, pancreatic pleural effusion, or cancer.
  Glucose is decreased with cancer, bacterial infections, or rheumatoid pleuritis.
  Pleural fluid pH is low in empyema (<7.2) and may be low in cancer.
    If cancer is suspected, the pleural fluid is sent for cytology. If cytology is negative, and cancer is still suspected, either a thoracoscopy, or needle biopsy of the pleura may be performed.
    The fluid is also sent for Gram staining and culture, and, if suspicious for tuberculosis, examination for TB markers (adenosine deaminase > 45 IU/L, interferon gamma > 140 pg/mL, or positive polymerase chain reaction (PCR) for tuberculous DNA).
  The most common causes of exudative pleural effusions are bacterial pneumonia, cancer (with lung cancer, breast cancer, and lymphoma causing approximately 75% of all malignant pleural effusions), viral infection, and pulmonary embolism.
  Other/ungrouped
  Other causes of pleural effusion include tuberculosis (though pleural fluid smears are rarely positive for AFB, this is the most common cause of pleural effusion in some developing countries), autoimmune disease such as systemic lupus erythematosus, bleeding (often due to chest trauma), chylothorax (most commonly caused by trauma), and accidental infusion of fluids.
  Less common causes include esophageal rupture or pancreatic disease, intra-abdominal abscess, rheumatoid arthritis, asbestos pleural effusion, Meigs syndrome (ascites and pleural effusion due to a benign ovarian tumor), and ovarian hyperstimulation syndrome.

Pleural effusions may also occur through medical/surgical interventions, including the use of medications (pleural fluid is usually eosinophilic), coronary artery bypass surgery, abdominal surgery, endoscopic variceal sclerotherapy, radiation therapy, liver or lung transplantation, and intra- or extravascular insertion of central lines.

Treatment

Treatment depends on the underlying cause of the pleural effusion.

Therapeutic aspiration may be sufficient; larger effusions may require insertion of an intercostal drain (either pigtail or surgical). When managing these chest tubes, it is important to make sure the chest tubes do not become occluded or clogged. A clogged chest tube in the setting of continued production of fluid will result in

residual fluid left behind when the chest tube is removed. This fluid can lead to complications such as hypoxia due to lung collapse from the fluid, or fibrothorax, later, when the space scars down. Repeated effusions may require chemical (talc, bleomycin, tetracycline/doxycycline), or surgical pleurodesis, in which the two pleural surfaces are scarred to each other so that no fluid can accumulate between them. This is a surgical procedure that involves inserting a chest tube, then either mechanically abrading the pleura or inse ting the chemicals to induce a scar. This requires the chest tube to stay in until the fluid drainage stops. This can take days to weeks and can require prolonged hospitalizations. If the chest tube becomes clogged, fluid will be left behind and the pleurodesis will fail.

CHAPTER FIFTEEN

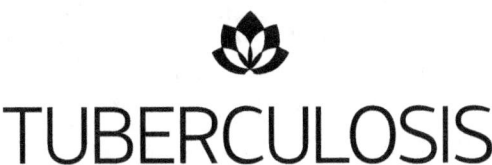

TUBERCULOSIS

Tuberculosis, MTB or TB (short for *tubercle bacillus*) is a common and in many cases lethal infectious disease caused by various strains of mycobacteria, usually *Mycobacterium tuberculosis*. Tuberculosis usually attacks the lungs but can also affect other parts of the body. It is spread through the air when people who have an active MTB infection cough, sneeze or otherwise transmit their saliva through the air. Most infections in humans result in asymptomatic, latent infection, and about one in ten latent infections eventually progresses to active disease, which, if left untreated, kills more than 50% of its victims.

The classic symptoms are a chronic cough with blood-tinged sputum, fever, night sweats, and weight loss (the last giving rise to the formerly prevalent colloquial term "consumption"). Infection of other organs causes a wide range of symptoms. Diagnosis relies on radiology (commonly chest X-rays), a tuberculin skin test, blood tests, as well as microscopic examination and microbiological culture of bodily fluids. Treatment is difficult and requires long courses of multiple antibiotics. Social contacts are also screened and treated if

necessary. Antibiotic resistance is a growing problem in (extensively) multi-drug-resistant tuberculosis. Prevention relies on screening programs and vaccination, usually with Bacillus Calmette-Guerin vaccine.

One-third of the world's population is thought to be infected with *M. tuberculosis*, and new infections occur at a rate of about one per second. The proportion of people who become sick with tuberculosis each year is stable or falling worldwide but, because of population growth, the absolute number of new cases is still increasing. In 2007 there were an estimated 13.7 million chronic active cases, 9.3 million new cases, and 1.8 million deaths, mostly in developing countries. In addition, more people in the developed world contract tuberculosis because their immune systems are more likely to be compromised due to higher exposure to immunosuppressive

drugs, substance abuse, or AIDS. The distribution of tuberculosis is not uniform across the globe; about 80% of the population in many Asian and African countries test positive in tuberculin tests, while only 5–10% of the US population test positive.

Signs and symptoms

When the disease becomes active, 75% of the cases involve infection in the lungs (pulmonary TB). Symptoms include chest pain, coughing up blood, and a productive, prolonged cough for more than three weeks. Systemic symptoms include fever, chills, night sweats, appetite loss, weight loss, pallor, and fatigue

In the other 25% of active cases, the infection moves from the lungs, causing other kinds of TB, collectively denoted extrapulmonary tuberculosis. This occurs more commonly in immunosuppressed persons and young children. Extrapulmonary infection sites include the pleura in tuberculous pleurisy, the central nervous

system in meningitis, the lymphatic system in scrofula of the neck, the genitourinary system in urogenital tuberculosis, and bones and joints in Pott's disease of the spine. An especially serious form is disseminated TB, more commonly known armillary tuberculosis. Extrapulmonary TB may co-exist with pulmonary TB.

Causes

The main cause of TB, *Mycobacterium tuberculosis* (MTB), is a small aerobic non-motile bacillus.

High lipid content of this pathogen accounts for many of its unique clinical characteristics. It divides every 16 to 20 hours, an extremely slow rate compared with other bacteria, which usually divide in less than an hour.

Since MTB has a cell wall but lacks a phospholipid outer membrane, it is classified as a Gram-positive bacterium. However, if a Gram stain is performed, MTB either stains very weakly Gram-positive or does not retain dye as a result of the high lipid &mycolic acid content of its cell wall. MTB can withstand weak disinfectants and survive in a dry state for weeks. In nature, the bacterium can grow only within the cells of a host organism, but *M. tuberculosis* can be cultured *in vitro*.

Using histological stains on expectorate samples from phlegm (also called sputum), scientists can identify MTB under a regular microscope. Since MTB retains certain stains after being treated with acidic solution, it is classified as an acid-fast bacillus (AFB). The most common acid-fast staining technique, the Ziehl-Neelsen stain, dyes AFBs a bright red that stands out clearly against a blue background. Other ways to visualize AFBs include an auramine-rhodamine stain and fluorescent microscopy.

The *M. tuberculosis* complex includes four other TB-causing mycobacteria: *M. bovis*, *M. africanum*, *M. canetti* and *M. microti*. *M. africanum* is not widespread, but in parts of Africa it is a significant cause of

tuberculosis. *M. bovis* was once a common cause of tuberculosis, but the introduction of pasteurized milk has largely eliminated this as a public health problem in developed countries. *M. canetti* is rare and seems to be limited to Africa, although a few cases have been seen in African emigrants. *M. microti* is mostly seen in immunodeficient people, although it is possible that the prevalence of this pathogen has been underestimated.

Other known pathogenic mycobacteria include *Mycobacterium leprae*, *Mycobacterium avium* and. *kansasii*. The latter two are part of the nontuberculous mycobacteria (NTM) group. Nontuberculous mycobacteria cause neither TB nor leprosy, but they *do* cause pulmonary diseases resembling TB.

Risk factors

People with silicosis have an approximately *30-fold* greater risk for developing TB. Silica particles irritate the respiratory system, causing immunogenic responses such as phagocytosis, which, as a consequence, results in high lymphatic vessel deposits It is this interference and blockage of macrophage function that increases the risk of tuberculosis. Persons with chronic renal failure and also on hemodialysis have an increased risk. Persons with diabetes mellitus have a risk for developing active TB that is two to four times greater than persons without diabetes mellitus, and this risk is likely to be greater in persons with insulin-dependent or poorly controlled diabetes. Other clinical conditions that have been associated with active TB include gastrectomy with attendant weight loss and malabsorption, jejunoileal bypass, renal and cardiac transplantation, carcinoma of the head or neck, and other neoplasms (e.g., lung cancer, lymphoma, and leukemia). Given that silicosis greatly increases the risk of tuberculosis, more research about the effect of various indoor or outdoor air pollutants on the disease would be necessary. Some possible indoor sources of silica include paint, concrete and Portland cement. Crystalline silica is found in concrete, masonry, sandstone, rock, paint, and other abrasives. The cutting, breaking, crushing, drilling, grinding, or abrasive blasting of these materials may produce fine silica dust. It can also be in soil, mortar, plaster, and shingles.

Low body weight is associated with risk of tuberculosis as well. A body mass index (BMI) below 18.5 increases the risk by 2–3 times. An increase in body weight lowers the risk. People with diabetes mellitus are at increased risk of contracting tuberculosis, and they have a poorer response to treatment, possibly due to poorer drug absorption.

Transmission

When people suffering from active pulmonary TB cough, sneeze, speak, sing, or spit, they expel infectious aerosol droplets 0.5 to 5 μm in diameter. A single sneeze can release up to 40,000 droplets. Each one of these droplets may transmit the disease, since the infectious dose of tuberculosis is very low and inhaling fewer than ten bacteria may cause an infection.

People with prolonged, frequent, or intense contact are at particularly high risk of becoming infected, with an estimated 22% infection rate. A person with active but untreated tuberculosis can infect 10–15 other people per year. Others at risk include people in areas where TB is common, people who inject illicit drugs, residents and employees of high-risk congregate settings, medically under-served and low-income populations, high-risk racial or ethnic minority populations, children exposed to adults in high-risk categories, those who are immunocompromised by conditions such as HIV/AIDS, people who take immunosuppressant drugs, and health care workers serving these high-risk clients.

Transmission can only occur from people with active—not latent—TB. The probability of transmission from one person to another depends upon the number of infectious droplets expelled by a carrier, the effectiveness of ventilation, the duration of exposure, and the virulence of the *m. tuberculosis* strain. The chain of transmission can be broken by isolating people with active disease and starting effective anti-tuberculous therapy. After two weeks of such treatment, people with non-resistant active TB generally cease to be contagious. If someone does become infected, then it will take three to four weeks before the newly infected person can transmit the disease to others.

Pathogenesis

About 90% of those infected with *Mycobacterium tuberculosis* have asymptomatic, latent TB infection (sometimes called LTBI), with only a 10% lifetime chance that a latent infection will progress to TB disease. However, if untreated, the death rate for these active TB cases is more than 50%.

TB infection begins when the mycobacteria reach the pulmonary alveoli, where they invade and replicate within the endosomes of alveolar macrophages. The primary site of infection in the lungs is called the Ghon focus, and is generally located in either the upper part of the lower lobe, or the lower part of the upper lobe. Bacteria are picked up by dendritic cells, which do not allow replication, although these cells can transport the bacilli to local (mediastinal) lymph nodes. Further spread is through the bloodstream to other tissues and organs where secondary TB lesions can develop in other parts of the lung (particularly the apex of the upper lobes), peripheral lymph nodes, kidneys, brain, and bone. All parts of the body can be affected by the disease, though it rarely affects the heart, skeletal muscles, pancreas and thyroid.

Tuberculosis is classified as one of the granulomatous inflammatory conditions. Macrophages, T lymphocytes, B lymphocytes and fibroblasts are among the cells that aggregate to form granulomas, with lymphocytes surrounding the infected macrophages. The granuloma prevents dissemination of the mycobacteria and provides a local environment for interaction of cells of the immune system. Bacteria inside the granuloma can become dormant, resulting in a latent infection. Another feature of the granulomas of human tuberculosis is the development of abnormal cell death (necrosis) in the centre of tubercles. To the naked eye this has the texture of soft white cheese and is termed caseous necrosis.

If TB bacteria gain entry to the bloodstream from an area of damaged tissue they spread through the body and set up many foci of infection, all appearing as tiny white tubercles in the tissues. This severe form of TB disease is most common in infants and the elderly and is called miliary tuberculosis. People with this disseminated TB have a fatality rate near 100% if untreated. However, if treated early, the fatality rate is reduced to about 10%.

In many people the infection waxes and wanes. Tissue destruction and necrosis are balanced by healing and fibrosis. The affected tissue is replaced by scarring and cavities filled with cheese-like white necrotic material. During active disease, some of these cavities are joined to the air passages bronchi and this material can be coughed up. It contains living bacteria and can, therefore, pass on the infection. Treatment with appropriate antibiotics kills bacteria and allows healing to take place. Upon cure, affected areas are eventually replaced by scar tissue.

If untreated, infection with *Mycobacterium tuberculosis* can cause lobar pneumonia.

Diagnosis

Tuberculosis is diagnosed definitively by identifying the causative organism (*Mycobacterium tuberculosis*) in a clinical sample (for example, sputum or pus). When this is not possible, a probable – although sometimes inconclusive– diagnosis may be made using imaging (X-rays or scans), a tuberculin skin test (Mantoux test) and/or an Interferon Gamma Release Assay (IGRA).

The main problem with tuberculosis diagnosis is the difficulty in culturing this slow-growing organism in the laboratory (it may take 4 to 12 weeks for blood or sputum culture). A complete medical evaluation for TB must include a medical history, a physical examination, a chest X-ray, microbiological smears, and cultures. It may also include a tuberculin skin test, a serological test. The interpretation of the tuberculin skin test depends upon the person's risk factors for infection and progression to TB diseases, such as exposure to other cases of TB or immunosuppression. Currently, latent infection is diagnosed in a non-immunized person by a tuberculin skin test, which yields a delayed hypersensitivity type response to an extract made from *M. tuberculosis*. Those immunized for TB or with the past-cleared infection will respond with delayed hypersensitivity parallel to those currently in a state of infection, so the test must be used with caution, particularly with regard to persons from countries where TB immunization is common. Tuberculin tests have the disadvantage of producing false negatives, especially when the person is co-morbid with sarcoidosis, Hodgkin's lymphoma, malnutrition, or most notably active tuberculosis disease. The newer interferon release assays (IGRAs) such as T-SPOT.TB and QuantiFERON-TB Gold in Tube overcome many of these problems. IGRAs are *in vitro* blood tests that are more specific than the skin test. IGRAs detect the release of interferon-gamma in response to mycobacterial proteins such as ESAT-6. These are not affected by immunization or environmental mycobacteria, so generate fewer false-positive results. There is also evidence that IGRAs are more sensitive than the skin test.

New TB tests have been developed that are fast and accurate. These include polymerase chain

reaction assays for the detection of bacterial DNA. One such molecular diagnostics test gives results in 100 minutes and is being currently offered to 116 low and middle-income countries at a discount with support from WHO and the Bill and Melinda Gates Foundation.

Another such test, which was approved by the FDA in 1996, is the amplified mycobacterium tuberculosis direct test (MTD, Gen-Probe). This test yields results in 2.5 to 3.5 hours, and it is highly sensitive and specific when used to test smears positive for acid-fast bacilli (AFB).

Screening

Mantoux tuberculin skin tests are often used for routine screening of high-risk individuals. Interferon-γ release assays are blood tests used in the diagnosis of some infectious diseases. There are currently two interferon-γ release assays available for the diagnosis of tuberculosis:

QuantiFERON-TB Gold (licensed in US, Europe and Japan); and

T-SPOT.TB, a form of ELISPOT (licensed in Europe).

Chest photofluorography has been used in the past for mass screening for tuberculosis.

Prevention

TB prevention and control takes two parallel approaches. In the first, people with TB and their contacts are identified and then treated. Identification of infections often involves testing high-risk groups for TB. In the second approach, children are vaccinated to protect them from TB. No vaccine is available that provides reliable protection for adults. However, in tropical areas where the levels of other species of mycobacteria are high, exposure to nontuberculous mycobacteria gives some protection against TB.

The World Health Organization (WHO) declared TB a global health emergency in 1993, and the Stop TB Partnership developed a Global Plan to Stop Tuberculosis that aims to save 14 million lives between 2006 and 2015. Since humans are the only host of *Mycobacterium tuberculosis*, eradication would be possible. This goal would be helped greatly by an effective vaccine.

Vaccines

Many countries use Bacillus Calmette-Guerin (BCG) vaccine as part of their TB control programmes, especially for infants. The BCG vaccine is one of the most widely used of all current vaccines, reaching >80% of neonates and infants in countries with a national vaccination schedule. One country that notably does not widely administer BCG is the United States, where TB is rather uncommon. BCG was the first vaccine for TB. From 1905, Albert Calmette and Camille Guérin worked at the Institute Pasteur de Lille and the Pasteur Institute in France developing BCG, administering the first human trials in 1921. However, deaths due to flawed manufacturing processes created public resistance to BCG, delaying mass vaccinations until after World War

The protective efficacy of BCG for preventing serious forms of TB (e.g. meningitis) in children is greater than 80%; its protective efficacy for preventing pulmonary TB in adolescents and adults varies by country (as low as 0% in South India for unknown reasons), but in the United Kingdom, its effectiveness exceeds 75%.

Infants or children with negative skin test results who are continually exposed to untreated or ineffectively treated people or will be continually exposed to multidrug-resistant TB.

Healthcare workers considered on an individual basis in settings in which a high percentage of MDR-TB has been found, the transmission of MDR-TB is likely, and TB control precautions have been implemented and were not successful.

BCG provides some protection against severe forms of pediatric TB, but has been shown to be unreliable against adult pulmonary TB, which accounts for most of the disease burden worldwide. Currently, there are more cases of TB on the planet than at any other time in history and most agree there is an urgent need for a newer, more effective vaccine that would prevent all forms of TB—including drug-resistant strains—in all age groups and among people with HIV.

Several new vaccines to prevent TB infection are being developed, among others by Aeras and TBVI. The first recombinant tuberculosis vaccine Mtb72F, entered clinical trials in the United States in 2004, sponsored by the National Institute of Allergy and Infectious Diseases (NIAID). A 2005 study showed that a DNA TB vaccine given with conventional chemotherapy can accelerate the disappearance of bacteria as well as protect against re-infection in mice; it may take four to five years to be available in humans. A very promising TB vaccine, MVA85A, is currently in phase II trials in South Africa by a group led by Oxford University, and is based on a genetically modified vaccinia virus. Many other strategies are also being used to develop novel vaccines, including both subunit vaccines (fusion molecules composed of two recombinant proteins delivered in an adjuvant) such as Hybrid-1, HyVac4 or M72, and recombinant adenoviruses such as Ad35. Some of these vaccines can be effectively administered without needles, making them preferable for areas where HIV is very common. All of these vaccines have been successfully tested in humans and are now in extended testing in TB-endemic regions. To encourage further discovery, researchers and policymakers are promoting new economic models of vaccine development including prizes, tax incentives and advance market commitments.

An experimental vaccine, with positive results in mouse models, may be effective in not only preventing infection, but also in eradicating the infection once established. A tuberculosis vaccine aimed at sterile *Mtb* eradication should be able to target latent *Mtb* as well as *Mtb* that causes early-stage tuberculosis. The vaccine is a combination of antigens Ag85B and ESAT-6 as well as the protein Rv2660c.

Ag85B and ESAT-6 together form the vaccine Hybrid-1, while Rv2660c is a protein that is expressed even in late-stage infections, when protein transcription is generally reduced. The novel combination of Ag85B, ESAT-6, and Rv2660c allows for both short- and long-term protection as a result of the continued expression of target proteins. The new vaccine, currently referred to as H56, works by promoting a polyfunctional CD4+ T cell response against tuberculosis protein components. Phase I clinical trials are scheduled to begin in Cape Town, South Africa in March 2011.

Treatment

Treatment for TB uses antibiotics to kill the bacteria. Effective TB treatment is difficult, due to the unusual structure and chemical composition of the mycobacterial cell wall, which makes many antibiotics ineffective and hinders the entry of drugs. The two antibiotics most commonly used are isoniazid and rifampicin. However, instead of the short course of antibiotics typically used to cure other bacterial infections, TB requires much longer periods of treatment (around 6 to 24 months) to entirely eliminate mycobacteria from the body. Latent TB treatment usually uses a single antibiotic, while active TB disease is best treated with combinations of several antibiotics, to reduce the risk of the bacteria developing antibiotic resistance. People with latent infections are treated to prevent them from progressing to active TB disease later in life.

Drug-resistant tuberculosis is transmitted in the same way as regular TB. Primary resistance occurs in persons infected with a resistant strain of TB. A person with fully susceptible TB develops secondary y resistance (acquired resistance) during TB therapy because of inadequate treatment, not taking the prescribed regimen appropriately, or using low-quality medication. Drug-resistant TB is a public health issue in many developing countries, as treatment is longer and requires more expensive drugs. Multi-drug-resistant tuberculosis (MDR-TB) is defined as resistance to the two most effective first-line TB drugs: rifampicin and isoniazid. Extensively drug-resistant TB (XDR-TB) is also resistant to three or more of the six classes of second-line drugs.

The DOTS (Directly Observed Treatment Short-course) strategy of tuberculosis treatment recommended by WHO was based on clinical trials done in the 1970s by Tuberculosis Research Centre, Chennai, India. The country in which a person with TB lives can determine what treatment they receive. This is because multidrug-resistant tuberculosis is resistant to most first-line medications, the use of second-line antituberculosis medications is necessary to cure the person. However, the price of these medications is high; thus, poor people in the developing world have no or limited access to these treatments.

In the early 1900s to 1950s doctors would try to collapse the infected lung by breaking several ribs or inflating that half of the chest with air.

Prognosis

Progression from TB infection to TB disease occurs when the TB bacilli overcome the immune system defenses and begin to multiply. In primary TB disease—1–5% of cases—this occurs soon after infection.

However, in the majority of cases, a latent infection occurs that has no obvious symptoms These dormant bacilli can produce tuberculosis in 2–23% of these latent cases, often many years after infection. The risk of reactivation increases with immunosuppression, such as that caused by infection with HIV. In people co-infected with *M. tuberculosis* and HIV, the risk of reactivation increases to 10% per year.

Studies utilizing DNA fingerprinting of *M. tuberculosis* strains have shown that reinfection contributes more substantially to recurrent TB than previously thought, with between 12% and 77% of cases attributable to reinfection (instead of reactivation).

Epidemiology

Roughly a third of the world's population has been infected with *M. tuberculosis*, and new infections occur at a rate of one per second. However, not all infections with *M. tuberculosis* cause TB disease and many infections are asymptomatic. n 2007, an estimated 13.7 million people had active TB disease, with 9.3 million new cases and 1.8

million deaths; the annual incidence rate varied from 363 per 100,000 in Africa to 32 per 100,000 in the Americas. Tuberculosis is the world's greatest infectious killer of women of reproductive age and the leading cause of death among people with HIV/AIDS. The rise in HIV infections and the neglect of TB control programs have enabled a resurgence of tuberculosis.[100] The emergence of drug-resistant strains has also contributed to this new epidemic with, from 2000 to 2004, 20% of TB cases being resistant to standard treatments and 2% resistant to second-line drugs. The rate at which new TB cases occur varies widely, even in neighboring countries, apparently because of differences in health care systems.

There are a number of known factors that make people more susceptible to TB infection: worldwide the most important of these is HIV. Co-infection with HIV is a particular problem in Sub-Saharan Africa, due to the high incidence of HIV in these countries. Smoking more than 20 cigarettes a day also increases the risk of TB by two to four times Diabetes mellitus is also an important risk factor that is growing in importance in developing countries. Other disease states that increase the risk of developing tuberculosis are Hodgkin lymphoma, end-stage renal disease, chronic lung disease, malnutrition, and alcoholism.

Diet may also modulate risk. For example, among immigrants in London from the Indian subcontinent, vegetarian Hindu Asians were found to have an 8.5-fold increased risk of tuberculosis, compared to Muslims who ate meat and fish daily. Although a causal link is not proved by this data, this increased risk could be caused by micronutrient deficiencies: possibly iron, vitamin B12 or vitamin D. Further studies have provided more evidence of a link between vitamin D deficiency and an increased risk of contracting tuberculosis Globally, the severe malnutrition common in parts of the developing world causes a large increase in the risk of developing active tuberculosis, due to its damaging effects on the immune system. Along with overcrowding, poor nutrition may contribute to the strong link observed between tuberculosis and poverty.

Prisoners, especially in poor countries, are particularly vulnerable to infectious diseases such as HIV/AIDS and TB. Prisons provide a condition that allows TB to spread rapidly, due to overcrowding, poor nutrition and a lack of health services. Since the early 1990s, TB outbreaks have been reported in prisons in many countries in Eastern Europe. The prevalence of TB in prisons is much higher than among the general population – in some countries as much as 40 times higher.

CHAPTER SIXTEEN

DYSPNEA, ASPHYXIA & HYPOXIA

Dyspnea

Shortness of breath (SOB), or air hunger, is the subjective symptom of *breathlessness*. It is a normal symptom of heavy exertion but becomes pathological if it occurs in unexpected situations. In 85% of cases it is due to either asthma, pneumonia, cardiac ischemia, interstitial lung disease, congestive heart failure, chronic obstructive pulmonary disease, or psychogenic causes. Treatment typically depends on the underlying cause.

Dyspnea does not have a well-defined or universally accepted definition. It is defined by the American Thoracic Society as the "subjective experience of breathing discomfort that consists of qualitatively distinct sensations that vary in intensity. The experience derives from interactions among multiple physiological, psychological, social, and environmental factors, and may induce secondary physiological and behavioral responses." Other definitions of dyspnea include "difficulty in breathing", "disordered or inadequate breathing "uncomfortable awareness of breathing simple "breathlessness". Acute breathlessness is defined as severe shortness of breath that develops over minutes to hours. Chronic breathlessness on the other hand comes on over weeks or months. Dyspnea is distinct from labored breathing, which is rather a common physical presentation of respiratory distress.

Differential diagnosis

While shortness of breath is generally caused by disorders of the cardiac or respiratory system other system such as neurological, musculoskeletal, endocrine, hematologic, and psychiatric may be the cause.

Diagnosis, an online medical expert system, listed 497 distinct causes in October 2010. The most common cardiovascular causes are acute myocardial infarction and congestive heart failure while common pulmonary causes include chronic obstructive pulmonary disease, asthma, pneumothorax, and pneumonia. On a pathophysiological basis the causes can be divided into: (1) an increased awareness of normal breathing such as during an anxiety attack, (2) an increase in the work of breathing and (3) an abnormality in the ventilatory system.

Acute coronary syndrome

Acute coronary syndrome frequently presents with retrosternal chest discomfort and difficulty catching the breath. It however may atypically present with shortness of breath alone. Risk factors include old age, smoking, hypertension, hyperlipidemia, and diabetes. An electrocardiogram and cardiac enzymes are important both for diagnosis and directing treatment. Treatment involves measures to decrease the oxygen requirement of the heart and efforts to increase blood flow.

Congestive heart failure

Congestive heart failure frequently presents with SOB with exertion, orthopnea, and paroxysmal nocturnal dyspnea. It affects between 1-2% of the general United States population and occurs in 10% of those over 65 years old. Risk factors for acute decompensation include high dietary salt intake, medication noncompliance, cardiac ischemia, dysrhythmias, renal failure, pulmonary emboli, hypertension, and infections. Treatment efforts are directed towards decreasing lung congestion.

Chronic obstructive pulmonary disease

People with chronic obstructive pulmonary disease (COPD), most commonly emphysema or chronic bronchitis, frequently have chronic shortness of breath and a chronic productive cough. An acute exacerbation presents with increased shortness of breath and sputum production. COPD is a risk factor for pneumothorax thus this condition should be ruled out. In an acute exacerbation treatment is with a combination of anticholinergics, beta$_2$-adrenoceptor agonists, steroids and possibly positive pressure ventilation.

Asthma

Asthma is the most common reason for presenting to the emergency with shortness of breath.]It is the most common lung disease in both developing and developed countries affecting about 5% of the population.

Other symptoms include wheezing, tightness in the chest, and a nonproductive cough Inhaled beta2-adrenergic agonist (salbutamol) are first line therapy and usually lead to prompt improvement.

Pneumothorax

Pneumothorax presents typically with pleuritic chest pain of acute onset and shortness of breath not improved with oxygen Physical findings may include absent breath sounds on one side of the chest, jugular venous distension, and tracheal deviation.

Pneumonia

The symptoms of pneumonia are fever, productive cough, shortness of breath, and pleuritic chest pain. Inspiratory crackles may be heard on exam. A chest x-ray can be useful to differential pneumonia from congestive heart failure. As the cause is usually a bacterial infections antibiotic are typically used for treatment.

Pulmonary embolism

Pulmonary embolism classically presents with an acute onset of shortness of breath Other presenting symptoms include pleuritic chest pain, cough, hemoptysis, and fever. Risk factors include deep vein thrombosis, recent surgery, cancer, and previous thromboembolism. It must always be considered in those with acute onset of shortness of breath due to its high risk of mortality. Diagnosis however may be difficult.[Treatment is typically with anticoagulants.

Other

Other important or common causes of shortness of breath include cardiac tamponade, anemia, anaphylaxis, interstitial lung disease and panic attacks. Cardiac tamponade presents with dyspnea, tachycardia, elevated jugular venous pressure, and pulsus paradoxus. The gold standard for diagnosis is ultrasound. Anemia, that develops gradually, usually presents with exertional dyspnea, fatigue, weakness, and tachycardia It may lead to heart failure. Anaphylaxis typically begins over a few minutes in a person with a previous history of the same. Other symptoms include urticaria, throat swelling, and gastrointestinal upset the primary treatment is epinephrine. Interstitial lung disease presents with gradual onset of shortness of breath typically with a history of a predisposing environmental exposure. Shortness of breath is often the only symptom in those with tachydysrhythmias. Panic attacks typically present with hyperventilation, sweating, and numbness. They are however a diagnosis of exclusion. Around 2/3 of women experience shortness of breath as a part of a normal pregnancy. Neurological conditions such as spinal cord injury, phrenic nerve injuries, Guillain-Barre syndrome, amyotrophic lateral sclerosis, multiple sclerosis and muscular dystrophy can all cause an individual to experience shortness of breath.

Pathophysiology

A number of different physiological pathway may lead to shortness of breath including via chemoreceptors, mechanoreceptors, and lung receptors.

It is currently thought that there are three main components that contribute to dyspnea: afferent signals, efferent signals, and central information processing. It is believed that the central processing in the brain compares the afferent and efferent signals, and that a "mismatch" results in the sensation of dyspnea. In other words, dyspnea may result when the need for ventilation (afferent signaling) is not being met by the physical breathing that is occurring (efferent signaling). Afferent signals are sensory neuronal signals that ascend to the brain. Afferent neurons significant in dyspnea arise from a large number of sources including the carotid bodies, medulla, lungs, and chest wall. Chemoreceptors in the carotid bodies and medulla supply information regarding the blood gas levels of O_2, CO_2 and H^+. In the lungs, juxtacapillary (J) receptors are sensitive to pulmonary interstitial edema, while stretch receptors signal bronchoconstriction. Muscle spindles in the chest wall signal the stretch and tension of the respiratory muscles. Thus, poor ventilation leading to hypercapnia, left heart failure leading to interstitial edema (impairing gas exchange), asthma causing bronchoconstriction (limiting airflow) and muscle fatigue leading to ineffective respiratory muscle action could all contribute to a feeling of dyspnea

Efferent signals are the motor neuronal signals descending to the respiratory muscles. The most important respiratory muscle is the diaphragm. Other respiratory muscles include the external and internal intercostal muscles, the abdominal muscles and the accessory breathing muscles.

As the brain receives its plentiful supply of afferent information relating to ventilation, it is able to compare it to the current level of respiration as determined by the efferent signals. If the level of respiration is inappropriate for the body's status then dyspnea might occur. It is worth noting that there is a psychological component of dyspnea as well, as some people may become aware of their breathing in such circumstances but not experience the distress typical of dyspnea.

The initial approach to evaluation begins by assessment of the airway, breathing, and circulation followed by a medical history and physical examination. Signs that represent significant severity include hypotension, hypoxemia, tracheal deviation, altered mental status, unstable dysrhythmia, stridor, intercostal indrawing, cyanosis, and absent breath sounds.

A number of scales may be used to quantify the degree of shortness of breath. It may be subjectively rated on a scale from 1 to 10 with descriptors associated with the number (The Modified Borg Scale). Alternatively, a scale such as the MRC Breathlessness Scale might be used - it suggests five different grades of dyspnea based on the circumstances in which it arises.

Blood tests

A number of labs maybe helpful in determining the cause of shortness of breath. D-dimer while useful to rule out a pulmonary embolism in those who are at low risk is not of much value if it is positive as it may be positive in a number of conditions that lead to shortness of breath. A low level of brain natriuretic peptide is useful in ruling out congestive heart failure however a high level while supportive of the diagnosis could also be due to advanced age, renal failure, acute coronary syndrome, or a large pulmonary embolism.

Imaging

A chest x-ray is useful to confirm or rule out a pneumothorax, pulmonary edema, or pneumonia.

Spiral computed tomography with intravenous radiocontrast is the imaging study of choice to evaluate for pulmonary embolism

Treatment

In those who are none palliative the primary treatment of shortness of breath is directed at its underlying cause. Extra oxygen is effective in those with hypoxia however has no effect in those with normal blood oxygen saturations even in those with who are palliative.

Physiotherapy

Individuals can benefit from a variety of physical therapy interventions. Persons with neurological/neuromuscular abnormalities may have breathing difficulties due to weak or paralyzed intercostal, abdominal and/or other muscles needed for ventilation. Some physical therapy interventions for this population include active assisted cough techniques, volume augmentation such as breath stacking, education about body position and ventilation patterns and movement strategies to facilitate breathing.

Palliative
Along with the measure above systemic immediate release opioids are beneficial in reducing the symptom of shortness of breath due to both cancer and non-cancer causes. There is a lack of evidence to recommend midazolam, nebulized opioids, the use of gas mixtures, or cognitive-behavioral therapy.

Asphyxia

Asphyxia or asphyxiation (from Greek *a-* "without" and σφύξις *asphyxia*, "heartbeat") is a condition of severely deficient supply of oxygen to the body that arises from being unable to breathe normally. An example of asphyxia is choking. Asphyxia causes generalized hypoxia, which primarily affects the tissues and organs. It can be caused by improper ventilation and charcoal burning in a closed room. Many incidents have been reported (death and coma).

Oxygen deficiency

The body creates the need to breathe from the excess carbon dioxide in the lungs; the body has no way to detect the absence of oxygen. Many gases, though non-toxic, are classified as simple asphyxiants in their pure form or in high concentrations for this very reason.

One form of asphyxiation is from entering a low oxygen atmosphere or an inert atmosphere, such as in a food oil tank that has a covering blanket of nitrogen or argon to shield the oil from atmospheric oxygen. Without sufficient oxygen to sustain life, people will act normally at first but will then abruptly feel dizzy and black out in a matter of seconds as the remaining oxygen in the blood stream is consumed. Oxygen deficient atmospheres are the basis for many occurrences of single and multiple deaths; the deceased will be found lying prone on the bottom of a tank, and then the observer will rush in to rescue them, and succumb to the same effect, hence the need to vent or purge the inert gases from all tanks before entry The use of simple asphyxiant gases, such as the inhalation of pure helium for entertainment purposes, has resulted in death and brain injury from oxygen deficiency. Other causes of oxygen deficiency include:

Carbon monoxide inhalation, such as from a car exhaust: carbon monoxide has a higher affinity than oxygen to the hemoglobin in the blood's red blood corpuscles, bonding with it tenaciously, and, in the process, displacing oxygen and preventing the blood from transporting oxygen around the body

Contact with certain chemicals, including pulmonary agents (such as phosgene) and blood agents (such as hydrogen cyanide)

Self-induced hypocapnia by hyperventilation, as in shallow water or deep-water blackout and the choking game

A seizure which stops breathing activity

Sleep apnea

Drug overdose

Ondine's curse, central alveolar hypoventilation syndrome, or primary alveolar hypoventilation, a disorder of the autonomic nervous system in which a patient must consciously breathe; although it is often said that persons with this disease will die if they fall asleep, this is not usually the case

Acute respiratory distress syndrome.

Exposure to extreme low pressure or vacuum to the pattern

Smothering-

Smothering is the mechanical obstruction of the flow of air from the environment into the mouth and/or nostrils, for instance, by covering the mouth and nose with a hand, pillow, or a plastic bag.]Smothering can be either partial or complete, where partial indicates that the person being smothered is able to inhale some air, although less than required. In a normal situation, smothering requires at least partial obstruction of both the nasal cavities and the mouth to lead to asphyxia. Smothering with the hands or chest is used in some combat sports to distract the opponent, and create openings for transitions, as the opponent is forced to react to the smothering.

In some cases, when performing certain routines, smothering is combined with simultaneous compressive asphyxia. One example is overlay, in which an adult accidentally rolls over an infant during co-sleeping, an accident that often goes unnoticed and is mistakenly thought to be sudden infant death syndrome. Other accidents involving a similar mechanism are cave-ins or when an individual is buried in sand or grain.

In homicidal cases, the term burking is often ascribed to a killing method that involves simultaneous smothering and compression of the torso. The term "burking" comes from the method William Burke and William Hare used to kill their victims during the West Port murders. They killed the usually-intoxicated victims by sitting on their chests and suffocating them by putting a hand over their nose and mouth, while using the other hand to push the victim's jaw up. The corpses had no visible injuries, and were supplied to medical schools for money.

This method is sometimes used by a lion to kill a buffalo, by opening its mouth over the buffalo's mouth and nostrils and securing itself with its canine teeth.

Compressive asphyxia

Compressive asphyxia (also called chest compression) is the mechanical limitation of the expansion of the lungs by compressing the torso, hence interfering with breathing.

Compressive asphyxia occurs when the chest or abdomen is compressed posteriorly. In accidents, the term traumatic asphyxia or crush asphyxia is usually used to describe compressive asphyxia resulting from being crushed or pinned under a large weight or force. An example of traumatic asphyxia includes cases in which an individual has been using acar-jack to repair a car from below, only to be crushed under the weight of the vehicle.

Pythons, anacondas, and other constrictor snakes kill through compressive asphyxia. In cases of co-sleeping ("overlay"), the weight of an adult or large child may compress an infant's chest, preventing proper expansion of the chest. Risk factors include large or obese adults, parental fatigue or impairment (sedation by drugs or alcohol) of the sleeping adult and small shared sleeping space (for example, both adult and infant sharing a couch).

In fatal crowd disasters, compressive asphyxia from being crushed against the crowd causes the large part of the deaths, rather than blunt trauma from trampling. This is what occurred at the Hillsborough Disaster in 1989, when 96 Liverpool fans were crushed to death in an overcrowded terrace. In confined spaces, people push and lean against each other; evidence from bent steel railings in several fatal crowd accidents have shown horizontal forces over 4500 N (equivalent to a weight of approximately 460 kg, or 1014 lbs.). In cases where people have stacked up on each other forming a human pile, estimations have been made of around 380 kg (838 lbs.) of compressive weight in the lowest layer.

The cause of death of the detainees who have been restrained and left prone, for example in police vehicles, and are not able to move into safer positions has been referred to as "positional asphyxia". "Restraint asphyxia" is a term used to describe the death of people who have died or lost consciousness (to die later in a coma from anoxic brain damage) while being restrained in positions that cause asphyxia by facial compression, neck compression or chest compression. Most occur during law enforcement or psychiatric restraint situations. It may be that the "positional asphyxia" deaths of detainees are actually active chest compression deaths caused by the weight of restrainers holding uncooperative detainees down in a prone position during the process of being handcuffed and otherwise secured. Thus, the passive deaths following custody restraint presumed to be due to positional asphyxia after being secured by mechanical restraints may actually be examples of active restraint asphyxia occurring during the process of placing restraints.

Chest compression is also featured in various grappling combat sports, where it is sometimes called wringing. Such techniques are used either to tire the opponent or as complementary or distractive moves in combination with pinning holds, or sometimes even as submission holds.

Perinatal asphyxia

Perinatal asphyxia is the medical condition resulting from deprivation of oxygen (hypoxia) to a newborn infant long enough to cause apparent harm. It results most commonly from a drop in maternal blood pressure or interference during delivery with blood flow to the infant's brain. This can occur due to inadequate circulation or perfusion, impaired respiratory effort, or inadequate ventilation. Perinatal asphyxia happens in 2 to 10 per 1000 newborns that are born at term

Nitrogen asphyxiation

Nitrogen asphyxiation is an occasional cause of accidental death and a theoretical method of capital punishment. The painful experience of suffocation is not caused by lack of oxygen, but rather because of a buildup of carbon dioxide in the bloodstream which is exhaled under normal circumstances. After just two or three breaths of pure nitrogen, the oxygen concentration in the lungs would be low enough for some oxygen already in the bloodstream to exchange back to the lungs and be eliminated by exhalation. Crude simulation of oxygen transport through the lungs and blood stream suggests that the partial pressure of oxygen in arterial blood would be about 50 percent of saturation 1 minute after switching gases and would reach zero within 3 minutes.

Hypoxia

Hypoxia, or hypoxia ion, is a pathological condition in which the body as a whole (generalized hypoxia) or a region of the body (tissue hypoxia) is deprived of adequate oxygen supply. Variations in arterial oxygen concentrations can be part of the normal physiology, for example, during strenuous physical exercise. A mismatch between oxygen supply and its demand at the cellular level may result in a hypoxic condition.

Hypoxia in which there is complete deprivation of oxygen supply is referred to as anoxia.

Hypoxia differs from hypoxemia in that, in the latter, the oxygen concentration within the arterial blood is abnormally low. It is possible to experience hypoxia and have a low oxygen content (e.g., due to anemia) but maintain high oxygen partial pressure (pO_2). Incorrect use of these terms can lead to confusion, especially as hypoxemia is among the causes of hypoxia (in hypoxemic hypoxia).

Generalized hypoxia occurs in healthy people when they ascend to high altitude, where it causes altitude sickness leading to potentially fatal complications: high altitude pulmonary edema (HAPE) and high-altitude cerebral edema (HACE). Hypoxia also occurs in healthy individuals when breathing mixtures of gases with a low oxygen content, e.g. while diving underwater especially when using closed-circuit rebreather systems that control the amount of oxygen in the supplied air. A mild and non-damaging intermittent hypoxia is used intentionally during altitude trainings to develop an athletic performance adaptation at both the systemic and cellular level.

Hypoxia is also a serious consequence of preterm birth in the neonate. The main cause for this is that the lungs of the human fetus are among the last organs to develop during pregnancy. To assist the lungs to distribute oxygenated blood throughout the body, infants at risk of hypoxia are often placed inside an incubator capable of providing continuous positive airway pressure (also known as a humid crib).

Classification

Hypoxemic hypoxia is a generalized hypoxia, an inadequate supply of oxygen to the body as a whole. The term "hypoxemic hypoxia" specifies hypoxia caused by low partial pressure of oxygen in arterial blood. In the other causes of hypoxia that follow, the partial pressure of oxygen in arterial blood is normal. Hypoxemic hypoxia may be due to:

Hypoventilation. Inadequate pulmonary minute ventilation (e.g., respiratory arrest or by drugs such as opiates)

Shunts in the pulmonary circulation or a right-to-left shunt in the heart. Shunts can be caused by collapsed alveoli that are still perfused or a block in ventilation to an area of the lung. Whatever the mechanism, blood meant for the pulmonary system is not ventilated and so no gas exchange occurs (the ventilation/perfusion ratio is decreased).

Normal anatomical shunt occurs due to Thebesian veins which empty into the left ventricle and the bronchial circulation which supplies the bronchi with oxygen.

Normal physiological shunts occur due to the effect of gravity. The highest concentration of blood in the pulmonary circulation occurs in the bases of the pulmonary tree compared to the highest pressure of gas in the apices of the lungs.

V/Q mismatch. When the ventilation does not match the perfusion through the parenchyma of the lung. This can occur for a variety of reasons, the commonest being a Pulmonary embolism

Diffusing defects such as pulmonary fibrosis where the Aa gradient has increased.

Decreased concentration of oxygen in inspired air. Low partial

pressure of atmospheric oxygen such as found at high altitude or by reduced replacement of oxygen in the breathing mix.

Low partial pressure of oxygen in the lungs when switching from inhaled anesthesia to atmospheric air, due to the Fink effect, or diffusion hypoxia.

Anemia in which arterial oxygen pressure is normal, but total oxygen content of the blood is reduced. This is due to a decreased total carrying capacity.

Hypoxia when the blood fails to deliver oxygen to target tissues.

Carbon monoxide poisoning which inhibits the ability of hemoglobin to release the oxygen bound to it.

Methemoglobinemia in which an abnormal version of hemoglobin accumulates in the blood

Histotoxic hypoxia in which quantity of oxygen reaching the cells is normal, but the cells are unable

to use the oxygen effectively, due to disabled oxidative phosphorylation enzymes. Cyanide toxicity is one example.

Signs and symptoms

The symptoms of generalized hypoxia depend on its severity and acceleration of onset. In the case of altitude sickness, where hypoxia develops gradually, the symptoms include headaches, fatigue, shortness of breath, a feeling of euphoria and nausea. In severe hypoxia, or hypoxia of very rapid onset, changes in levels of consciousness, seizures, coma, priapism, and death occur. Severe hypoxia induces a blue discoloration of the skin, called cyanosis. Because hemoglobin is a darker red when it is not bound to oxygen (deoxyhemoglobin), as opposed to the rich red color that it has when bound to oxygen (oxyhemoglobin), when seen through the skin it has an increased tendency to reflect blue light back to the eye. In cases where the oxygen is displaced by another molecule, such as carbon monoxide, the skin may appear 'cherry red' instead of cyanotic.

Pathophysiology

After mixing with water vapor and expired CO_2 in the lungs, oxygen diffuses down a pressure gradient to enter arterial blood where its partial pressure is around 100 mmHg (13.3 kPa). Arterial blood flow delivers oxygen to the peripheral tissues, where it again diffuses down a pressure gradient into the cells and into their mitochondria. These bacteria-like cytoplasmic structures strip hydrogen from fuels (glucose, fats and some amino acids) to burn with oxygen to form water. The fuel's carbon is oxidized to CO_2, which diffuses down its partial pressure gradient out of the cells into venous blood to be exhaled finally by the lungs.

Experimentally, oxygen diffusion becomes rate limiting (and lethal) when arterial oxygen partial pressure falls to 40 mmHg (5.3 kPa) or below.

If oxygen delivery to cells is insufficient for the demand (hypoxia), hydrogen will be shifted to pyruvic

acid converting it to lactic acid. This temporary measure (anaerobic metabolism) allows small amounts of energy to be produced. Lactic acid builds up (in tissues and blood) is a sign of inadequate mitochondrial oxygenation, which may be due to hypoxemia, poor blood flow (e.g., shock) or a combination of both. If severe or prolonged it could lead to cell death.

Vasoconstriction and vasodilation

In most tissues of the body, the response to hypoxia is vasodilation. By widening the blood vessels, the tissue allows greater perfusion.

By contrast, in the lungs, the response to hypoxia is vasoconstriction. This is known as "Hypoxic pulmonary vasoconstriction", or "HPV".

Treatment

To counter the effects of high-altitude diseases, the body must return arterial pO_2 toward normal. Acclimatization, the means by which the body adapts to higher altitudes, only partially restore es pO_2 to standard levels. Hyperventilation, the body's most common response to high-altitude conditions, increases alveolar pO_2 by raising the depth and rate of breathing. However, while pO_2 does improve with hyperventilation, it does not return to normal. Studies of miners and astronomers working at 3000 meters and above show improved alveolar pO_2 with full acclimatization, yet the pO_2 level remains equal to or even below the threshold for continuous oxygen therapy for patients with chronic obstructive pulmonary disease (COPD). In addition, there are complications involved with acclimatization. Polycythemia, in which the body increases the number of red blood cells in circulation, thickens the blood, raising the danger that the heart can't pump it.

In high-altitude conditions, only oxygen enrichment can counteract the effects of hypoxia. By increasing the concentration of oxygen in the air, the effects of lower barometric pressure are countered and the level of arterial pO_2 is restored toward normal capacity. A small amount of supplemental oxygen reduces the equivalent altitude in climate-controlled rooms. At 4000 m, raising the oxygen concentration level by 5 per cent via an oxygen concentrator and an existing ventilation system provides an altitude equivalent of 3000 m, which is much more tolerable for the increasing number of low-landers who work in high altitude In a study of astronomers working in Chile at 5050 m, oxygen concentrators increased the level of oxygen concentration by almost 30 percent (that is, from 21 percent to 27 percent). This resulted in increased worker productivity, less fatigue, and improved sleep.

Oxygen concentrators are uniquely suited for this purpose. They require little maintenance and electricity, provide a constant source of oxygen, and eliminate the expensive, and often dangerous, task of transporting oxygen cylinders to remote areas. Offices and housing already have climate-controlled rooms, in which temperature and humidity are kept at a constant level. Oxygen can be added to this system easily and relatively cheaply.

CHAPTER SEVENTEEN

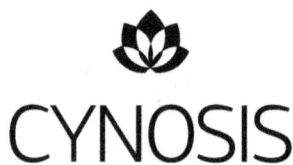

CYNOSIS

Cyanosis is the appearance of a blue or purple coloration of the skin or mucous membranes due to the tissues near the skin surface being low on oxygen. The onset of cyanosis is 2.5 g/dL of deoxyhemoglobin. The bluish color is more readily apparent in those with high hemoglobin counts than it is ith those with anemia. Also, the bluer color is more difficult to detect on deeply pigmented skin. When signs of cyanosis first appear, such as on the lips or fingers, intervention should be made within 3–5 minutes because a severe hypoxia or severe circulatory failure has induced the cyanosis.

The name *cyanosis*, literally means "the blue disease" or "the blue condition". It is derived from the color cyan, which comes from *kyanos*, the Greek word for blue.

Human blood is always a shade of red, and the more oxygenated the blood the brighter the shade of red. The more deoxygenated the blood, the darker red it is within the blood vessels, and the more bluish it appears on the skin. This color shift occurs because the optical properties of skin shift the darker red colors towards the bluer. (Some colors are refracted and absorbed more than others.) A similar phenomenon makes the sky appear blue.

Cyanosis is defined as a bluish discoloration, especially of the skin and mucous membranes due to excessive concentration of deoxyhemoglobin in the blood.

Differential diagnosis

Cyanosis is divided in to two main types: central (around the core and lips) and peripheral (only the extremities are affected). Cyanosis can occur in the fingers, including underneath the fingernails, as well as other extremities (called peripheral cyanosis), or in the lips and tongue (central cyanosis).

Central cyanosis

Central cyanosis is often due to a circulatory or ventilatory problem that leads to poor blood oxygenation in the lungs. It develops when arterial saturation of blood with oxygen is ≤85%. Cyanosis may not be detected until saturation is 75% in dark-skinned individuals.

Acute cyanosis can be a result of asphyxiation or choking, and is one of the surest signs that respiration is being blocked.

Causes

Central Nervous System:
    Intracranial hemorrhage
    Cerebral anoxia
    Drug overdose (e.g. Heroin)
    Respiratory System:
    Bronchiolitis
    Bronchospasm (e.g. Asthma)
    Lung disease

Pulmonary embolism
Hypoventilation
COPD (emphysema and chronic bronchitis)
Cardiac Disorders:
>   Congenital heart disease (e.g. Tetralogy of Fallot, right to left shunts in heart or great vessels)

Heart failure
Heart valve disease
Myocardial infarction
Blood:
Methemoglobinemia
Polycythemia
Others:
High altitude
Hypothermia

Congenital cyanosis (HbM Boston) arises from a mutation in the α-codon which results in a change of primary sequence, H →Y. Tyrosine stabilizes the Fe (III) form (oxyhemoglobin) creating a permanent T-state of Hb.

Obstructive sleep apnea
Peripheral cyanosis

Peripheral cyanosis is the blue tint in fingers or extremities, due to inadequate circulation. The blood reaching the extremities is not oxygen rich and when viewed through the skin a combination of factors can lead to the appearance of a blue colour. All factors contributing to central cyanosis can also cause peripheral symptoms to appear, however peripheral cyanosis can be observed without there being heart or lung failures. Small blood vessels may be restricted and can be treated by increasing the normal oxygenation level of the blood.

Causes

All common causes of central cyanosis
Arterial obstruction
Cold exposure (due to vasoconstriction)
Raynaud's phenomenon (vasoconstriction)
Reduced cardiac output (e.g. heart failure, hypovolemia)
Vasoconstriction
Venous obstruction (e.g. deep vein thrombosis)
Differential cyanosis

Differential cyanosis is the bluish coloration of the lower but not the upper extremity and the head. This is seen in patients with a patent ductus arteriosus. Patients with a large ductus develop progressive pulmonary vascular disease, and pressure overload of the right ventricle occurs. As soon as pulmonary pressure exceeds aortic pressure, shunt reversal (right-to-left shunt) occurs. The upper extremity remains pink because the brachiocephalic trunk, left common carotid trunk and the left subclavian trunk is given off proximal to the PDA.

CHAPTER EIGHTEEN

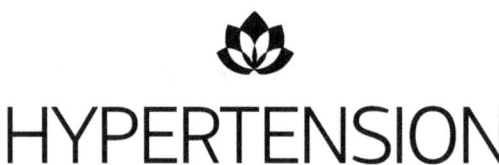

HYPERTENSION

Hypertension (HTN) or high blood pressure is a cardiac chronic medical condition in which the systemic arterial blood pressure is elevated. It is the opposite of hypotension. Hypertension is classified as either primary (essential) hypertension or secondary hypertension; About 90–95% of cases are categorized as "primary hypertension," which means high blood pressure with no obvious medical cause. The remaining 5–10% of cases (Secondary hypertension) are caused by other conditions that affect the kidneys, arteries, heart or endocrine system. Persistent hypertension is one of the risk factors for stroke, myocardial infarction, heart failure and arterial aneurysm, and is a leading cause of chronic kidney failure. Moderate elevation of arterial blood pressure leads to shortened life expectancy. Dietary and lifestyle changes can improve blood pressure control and decrease the risk of associated health complications, although drug treatment may prove necessary in patients for whom lifestyle changes prove ineffective or insufficient.

Classification

Blood pressure is usually classified based on the systolic and diastolic blood pressures. Systolic blood pressure is the blood pressure in vessels during a heartbeat. Diastolic blood pressure is the pressure between heartbeats. A systolic or the diastolic blood pressure measurement higher than the accepted normal values for the age of the individual is classified as prehypertension or hypertension.

Hypertension has several sub-classifications including, hypertension stage I, hypertension stage II, and isolated systolic hypertension.

Isolated systolic hypertension refers to elevated systolic pressure with normal diastolic pressure and is common in the elderly. These classifications are made after averaging a patient's resting blood pressure readings taken on two or more office visits. Individuals older than 50 years are classified as having hypertension if their blood pressure is consistently at least 140 mmHg systolic or 90 mmHg diastolic. Patients with blood pressures higher than 130/80 mmHg with concomitant presence of diabetes mellitus or kidney disease require further treatment. Hypertension is also classified as resistant if medications do not reduce blood pressure to normal levels.

Exercise hypertension is an excessively high elevation in blood pressure during exercise. The range considered normal for systolic values during exercise is between 200- and 230-mm Hg.[10]Exercise hypertension may indicate that an individual is at risk for developing hypertension at rest.

Signs and symptoms
Mild to moderate essential hypertension is usually asymptomatic.
Accelerated hypertension
Accelerated hypertension is associated
with headache, drowsiness, confusion, vision disorders, nausea, and vomiting. These symptoms are collectively called hypertensive encephalopathy. Hypertensive encephalopathy is caused by severe small blood vessel congestion and brain swelling, which is reversible if blood pressure is lowered.

Secondary hypertension
Some additional signs and symptoms suggest that the hypertension is caused by disorders in hormone regulation. Hypertension combined with obesity distributed on the trunk of the body, accumulated fat on the back of the neck ('buffalo hump'), wide purple marks on the abdomen (abdominal striae), or the recent onset of diabetes suggests that an individual has a hormone disorder known as Cushing's syndrome. Hypertension caused by other hormone disorders such as hyperthyroidism, hypothyroidism, or growth hormone excess will be accompanied by additional symptoms specific to these disorders. For example, hyperthyroidism can cause weight loss, tremors, heart rate abnormalities, reddening of the palms, and increased sweating. Signs and symptoms associated with growth hormone excess include coarsening of facial features, protrusion of the lower jaw, enlargement of the tongue, excessive hair growth, darkening of the skin color, and excessive sweating. Other hormone disorders

like hyperaldosteronism may cause fewer specific symptoms such as numbness, excessive urination, excessive sweating, electrolyte imbalances and dehydration, and elevated blood alkalinity. and also cause mental pressure.

In pregnancy

Hypertension in pregnant women is one symptom of pre-eclampsia.

Pre-eclampsia can progress to a life-threatening condition called eclampsia, which is the development of protein in the urine, generalized swelling, and severe seizures. Other symptoms indicating that brain function is becoming impaired may precede these seizures such as nausea, vomiting, headaches, and vision loss. In addition, the systemic vascular resistance and blood pressure decrease during pregnancy. The body must compensate by increasing cardiac output and blood volume to provide sufficient circulation in the utero-placental arterial bed.

In children

Some signs and symptoms are especially important in newborns and infants such as failure to

thrive, seizures, irritability, lack of energy, and difficulty breathing. In children, hypertension can cause headache, fatigue, blurred vision, nosebleeds, and facial paralysis.

Even with the above clinical symptoms, the true incidence of pediatric hypertension is not known. In adults, hypertension has been defined due to the adverse effects caused by hypertension. However, in children, similar studies have not been performed thoroughly to link any adverse effects with the increase in blood pressure. Therefore, the prevalence of pediatric hypertension remains unknown due to the lack of scientific knowledge.

Causes

Essential hypertension

Essential hypertension is the most prevalent hypertension type, affecting 90–95% of hypertensive patients. Although no direct cause has been identified, there are many factors such as sedentary lifestyle, smoking, stress, visceral obesity, potassium deficiency (hypokalemia), obesity (more than 85% of cases occur in those with a body mass index greater than 25), salt (sodium)

sensitivity, alcohol intake, and vitamin D deficiency that increase the risk of developing hypertension. Risk also increases with ageing, some inherited genetic mutations and having a family history of hypertension. An elevated level of renin, a hormone secreted by the kidney, is another risk factor, s is the sympathetic nervous system overactivity. Insulin resistance, which is a component of syndrome X (or the metabolic syndrome), is also thought to contribute to hypertension. Recent studies have implicated low birth weight as a risk factor for adult essential hypertension.

Secondary hypertension

Secondary hypertension by definition results from an identifiable cause. This type is important to recognize since it's treated differently to essential hypertension, by treating the underlying cause of the elevated blood pressure. Hypertension results in the compromise or imbalance of the pathophysiological mechanisms, such as the hormone-regulating endocrine system, that regulate blood plasma volume and heart function. Many conditions cause hypertension.

Some are common, well-recognized secondary causes such

As Cushing's syndrome, which is a condition where the adrenal glands overproduce the hormone cortisol. Hypertension is also caused by other conditions that cause hormone changes, such as hyperthyroidism, hypothyroidism (citation needed), and certain tumors of the adrenal medulla (e.g., pheochromocytoma). Other common causes of secondary hypertension include kidney disease, obesity/metabolic disorder, pre-eclampsia during pregnancy, the congenital defect known as coarctation of the aorta, and certain prescription and illegal drugs.

Pathophysiology

Most of the mechanisms associated with secondary hypertension are generally fully understood. However, those associated with essential (primary) hypertension are far less understood. What is known is

that cardiac output is raised early in the disease course, with total peripheral resistance (TPR) normal; over time cardiac output drops to normal levels but TPR is increased. Three theories have been proposed to explain this:

Inability of the kidneys to excrete sodium, resulting in natriuretic factors such as Atrial Natriuretic Factor being secreted to promote salt excretion with the side effect of raising total peripheral resistance.

An overactive Renin-angiotensin system leads to vasoconstriction and retention of sodium and water. The increase in blood volume plus vasoconstriction leads to hypertension.

An overactive sympathetic nervous system, leading to increased stress responses.

It is also known that hypertension is highly heritable and polygenic (caused by more than one gene) and a few candidate genes have been postulated in the etiology of this condition.

Recently, work related to the association between essential hypertension and sustained endothelial damage has gained popularity among hypertension scientists. It remains unclear however whether endothelial changes precede the development of hypertension or whether such changes are mainly due to long standing elevated blood pressures.

Diagnosis

Hypertension is generally diagnosed on the basis of a persistently high blood pressure. Usually this requires three separate sphygmomanometers (see figure) measurements at least one week apart. Often, this entails three separate visits to the physician's office. Initial assessment of the hypertensive patient should include a complete history and physical examination. Exceptionally, if the elevation is extreme, or if symptoms of organ damage are present then the diagnosis may be given and treatment started immediately.

Once the diagnosis of hypertension has been made, physicians will attempt to identify the underlying cause based on risk factors and other symptoms, if present. Secondary hypertension is more common in preadolescent children, with most cases caused by renal disease. Primary or essential hypertension is more common in adolescents and has multiple risk factors, including obesity and a family history of hypertension. Laboratory tests can also be performed to identify possible causes of secondary hypertension, and determine if hypertension has caused damage to the heart, eyes, and kidneys.

Additional tests for Diabetes and high cholesterol levels are also

usually performed because they are additional risk factors for the development of heart disease require treatment. Tests typically performed are classified as follows:

Creatinine (renal function) testing is done to determine if kidney disease is present, which can be either the cause or result of hypertension. In addition, it provides a baseline measurement of kidney function that can be used to monitor for side-effects of certain antihypertensive drugs on kidney function. Additionally, testing of urine samples for protein is used as a secondary indicator of kidney disease. Glucose testing is done to determine if diabetes mellitus is present. Electrocardiogram (EKG/ECG) testing is done to check for evidence of the heart being under strain from high blood pressure. It may also show if there is thickening of the heart muscle (left ventricular hypertrophy) or has experienced a prior minor heart disturbance such as a silent heart attack. A chest X-ray may be performed to look for signs of heart enlargement or damage to heart tissue.

Prevention

The degree to which hypertension can be prevented depends on a number of features including current blood pressure level, sodium/potassium balance, detection and omission of environmental toxins, changes in end/target organs (retina, kidney, heart, among others), risk factors for cardiovascular diseases and the age at diagnosis of prehypertension or at risk for hypertension. A prolonged assessment that involves repeated blood pressure measurements provides the most accurate blood pressure level assessment.

Following this, lifestyle changes are recommended to lower blood pressure, before the initiation of prescription drug therapy. The process of managing prehypertension according the guidelines of the British Hypertension Society suggest the following lifestyle changes:

Weight reduction and regular aerobic exercise (e.g., walking): Regular exercise improves blood flow and helps to reduce the resting heart rate and blood pressure.[47]

Reduce dietary sugar

Reduce sodium (salt) in the body by disuse of condiment sodium and the adoption of a high potassium diet which rids

the renal system of excess sodium. Many people use potassium chloride salt substitute to reduce their salt intake.

Additional dietary changes beneficial to reducing blood pressure include the DASH diet (dietary approaches to stop hypertension) which is rich in fruits and vegetables and low-fat or fat-free dairy products. Research sponsored by the National Heart, Lung, and Blood Institute. showed this diet to be effective. In addition, an increase in dietary potassium, which offsets the effect of sodium has been shown highly effective in reducing blood pressure. Discontinuing tobacco use and alcohol consumption has been shown to lower blood pressure. The exact mechanisms are not fully understood, but blood pressure (especially systolic) always transiently increases following alcohol or nicotine consumption.

Abstaining from cigarette smoking reduces the risks of stroke and heart attack associated with hypertension.

Vasodilators such as niacin.

Limiting alcohol intake to less than 2 standard drinks per day can reduce systolic blood pressure by between 2-4mmHg.

Reducing stress, for example with relaxation therapy, such as meditation and other Mindbody relaxation techniques, by reducing environmental stress such as high sound levels and over- illumination can also lower blood pressure. Jacobson's Progressive Muscle Relaxation and biofeedback are also beneficial, such as device-guided paced breathing,

although meta-analysis suggests it is not effective unless combined with other relaxation techniques. Increasing omega 3 fatty acids can help lower hypertension. Fish oil is shown to lower blood pressure in hypertensive individuals. The fish oil may increase sodium and water excretion.

Treatment

Lifestyle modifications

The first line of treatment for hypertension—which are the same as the recommended preventative lifestyle changes— include:

Dietary changes
Physical exercise
Weight loss

These have all been shown to significantly reduce blood pressure in people with hypertension. If hypertension is high enough to justify immediate use of medications, lifestyle changes are still recommended in conjunction with medication. Drug prescription should take into account the patient's absolute cardiovascular risk (including risk of myocardial infarction and stroke) as well as blood pressure readings, in order to gain a more accurate picture of the patient's cardiovascular profile. Different programs aimed to reduce psychological stress such as biofeedback, relaxation or meditation are dvertised to reduce hypertension. However, in general claims of efficacy are not supported by scientific studies, which have been in general of low quality.

Regarding dietary changes, a low sodium diet is beneficial;

Medications

Several classes of medications, collectively referred to as antihypertensive drugs, are currently available for treating hypertension. Reduction of the blood pressure by 5 mmHg can decrease the risk of stroke by 34%, of ischemic heart disease by 21%, and reduce the likelihood of dementia, heart failure, and mortality from cardiovascular disease. The aim of treatment should be to reduce blood pressure to <140/90 mmHg for most individuals, and lower for individuals with diabetes or kidney disease (some medical professionals recommend keeping levels below 120/80 mmHg). If the blood pressure goal is not met, a change in treatment should be made as therapeutic inertia is a clear impediment to blood pressure control. Comorbidity also plays a role in determining target blood pressure, with lower BP targets applying to patients with end-organ damage or proteinuria.

The first line antihypertensive supported by the best evidence is a low dose thiazide-based diuretic.

Often multiple medications are needed to be combined to achieve the goal blood pressure. Commonly used prescription drugs include: ACE inhibitors, alpha blockers, angiotensin II receptor antagonists, beta blockers, calcium channel blockers, diuretics (e.g. hydrochlorothiazide), direct renin inhibitors.

Some examples of common combined prescription drug treatments include:

A fixed combination of an ACE inhibitor and a calcium channel blocker. One example of this is the combination of perindopril and amlodipine, the efficacy of which has been demonstrated in individuals with glucose intolerance or metabolic syndrome.

A fixed combination of a diuretic and an ARB.

Combinations of an ACE inhibitor or angiotensin II–receptor antagonist, a diuretic and an NSAID (including selective COX-2 inhibitors and non-prescribed drugs such as ibuprofen) should be avoided whenever possible due to a high documented risk of acute renal failure. The combination is known colloquially as a "triple whammy" in the Australian health industry.

In the elderly

Treating moderate to severe high blood pressure decreases death rates in those under 80 years of age. In those over 80 years old there was a decrease in morbidity but no decrease in mortality. The recommended BP goal is <140/90 mm Hg with thiazide diuretics being the first line medication.

Complications

Hypertension is the most important risk factor for death in industrialized countries It increases hardening of the arteries thus predisposes individuals to heart disease, peripheral vascular disease, and strokes. Types of heart disease that may occur include: myocardial infarction, heart failure, and left ventricular hypertrophy Other complications include:

Hypertensive retinopathy

Hypertensive nephropathy

If blood pressure is very high hypertensive encephalopathy may result.

Silent stroke is a type of stroke (infarct) that does not have any outward symptoms (asymptomatic), and the patient is typically unaware they have suffered a stroke. Despite not causing identifiable symptoms a silent stroke still causes damage to the brain, and places the patient at increased risk for a major stroke in the future. Hypertension is the major treatable risk factor associated with silent stokes.

Epidemiology

In the year 2000 it is estimated that nearly one billion people or ~26% of the adult population had hypertension worldwide. It was common in both developed (333 million) and undeveloped (639 million) countries.

However, rates vary markedly in different regions with rates as low as 3.4% (men) and 6.8% (women) in rural India and as high as 68.9% (men) and 72.5% (women) in Poland.

In 1995 it is estimated that 43 million people in the United States had hypertension or were taking antihypertensive medication, almost 24% of the adult population. The prevalence of hypertension in the United States is increasing and reached 29% in 2004. It is more common in blacks and native Americans and less in whites and Mexican Americans, rates increase with age, and is greater in the southeastern United States. Hypertension is more prevalent in men (though menopause tends to decrease this difference) and those of low socioeconomic status. Over 90–95% of adult hypertension

is essential hypertension. The most common cause of secondary hypertension is primary aldosteronism. The incidence of exercise hypertension is reported to range from 1–10%.

In children

The prevalence of high blood pressure in the young is increasing. Most childhood hypertension, particularly in preadolescents, is secondary to an underlying disorder. Kidney disease is the most common (60–70%) cause of hypertension in

children. Adolescents usually have primary or essential hypertension, which accounts for 85–95% of cases.

Defibrillation

Defibrillation is a common treatment for life-threatening cardiac arrhythmias, ventricular fibrillation and pulseless ventricular tachycardia. Defibrillation consists of delivering a therapeutic dose of electrical energy to the affected heart with a device called a defibrillator. This depolarizes a critical mass of the heart muscle, terminates the arrhythmia, and allows normal sinus rhythm to be reestablished by the body's natural pacemaker, in the sinoatrial node of the heart. Defibrillators can be external, transvenous, or

implanted, depending on the type of device used or needed. Some external unnits, known as automated external defibrillators (AEDs), automate the diagnosis of treatable rhythms, meaning that lay responders or bystanders are able to use them successfully with little, or in some cases no training at all.

History

Defibrillation was first demonstrated in 1899 by Jean-Louis Prevost and Frederic Batelli, two physiologists from University of Geneva, Switzerland. They discovered that small electric shocks could induce ventricular fibrillation in dogs, and that larger charges would reverse the condition.

In 1933 a Dr Albert Hyman a heart specialist at the Beth Davis Hospital of New York city and a C. Henry Hyman, an electrical engineer, looking for an alternative to injecting powerful drugs directly into the heart, came up with an invention that used an electrical shock in place of drug injection. This invention was called the *Hyman Otor* where a hollow needle is used to pass an insulated wire to the heart area to deliver the electrical shock. The hollow steel needle being one end of the circuit and the insulated wire the other end. Whether the *Hyman Otor* was a success is unknown. The first use on a human was in 1947 by Claude Beck professor of surgery at Case Western Reserve University. Beck's theory was that ventricular fibrillation often occurred in hearts which were fundamentally healthy, in his terms "Hearts that are too good to die", and that there must be a way of saving them. Beck first used the technique successfully on a 14-year-old boy who was being operated on for a congenital chest defect. The boy's chest was surgically opened, and manual cardiac massage was undertaken for 45 minutes until the arrival of the defibrillator. Beck used internal paddles on either side of the heart, along with procainamide, an antiarrhythmic drug, and achieved return of normal sinus rhythm.

These early defibrillators used the alternating current from a power socket, transformed from the 110-240 volts available in the line, up to between 300 and 1000 volts, to the exposed heart by way of 'paddle' type electrodes. The technique was often ineffective in reverting VF while morphological studies showed damage to the cells of the heart muscle post mortem. The nature of the AC machine with a large transformer also made these units very hard to transport, and they tended to be large units on wheels.

Closed-chest method

Until the early 1950s, defibrillation of the heart was possible only when the chest cavity was open during surgery. The technique used an alternating current from a 300 or greater volt source delivered to the sides of the exposed heart by 'paddle' electrodes where

each electrode was a flat or slightly concave metal plate of about 40 mm diameter. The closed-chest defibrillator device which applied an alternating current of greater than 1000 volts, conducted by means of externally applied electrodes through the chest cage to the heart, was pioneered by Dr V. Skin with assistance by A. Klimov in Frunze, USSR (today known as Bishkek, Kyrgyzstan) in the mid-1950s

Move to direct current

In 1959 Bernard Lown commenced research into an alternative technique which involved charging of a bank of capacitors to approximately 1000 volts with an energy content of 100-200 joules then delivering the charge through an inductance such as to produce a heavily damped sinusoidal wave of finite duration (~5milliseconds) to the heart by way of paddle electrodes. The work of lown was taken to clinical application by engineer Barouh Berkovits with his "cardioverter".

The Lown waveform, as it was known, was the standard for defibrillation until the late 1980s when numerous studies showed that a biphasic truncated waveform (BTE) was equally efficacious while requiring the delivery of lower levels of energy to produce defibrillation. A side effect was a significant reduction in weight of the machine. The BTE waveform, combined with automatic measurement of transthoracic impedance is the basis for modern defibrillators.

Portable units become available

A major breakthrough was the introduction of portable defibrillators used out of the hospital. This was pioneered in the early 1960s by Prof. Frank Pantridge in Belfast. Today portable defibrillators are among the many very important tools carried by ambulances.

They are the only proven way to resuscitate a person who has had a cardiac arrest unwitnessed by EMS who is still in persistent ventricular fibrillation or ventricular tachycardia at the arrival of pre-hospital providers.

Gradual improvements in the design of defibrillators, partly based on the work developing implanted versions (see below), have led to the availability of Automated External Defibrillators. These devices can analyses the heart rhythm by themselves, diagnose the shockable rhythms, and charge to treat. This means that no clinical skill is required in their use, allowing lay people to respond to emergencies effectively.

Change to a biphasic waveform Until the late 1980s, external defibrillators delivered a Lown type waveform (see Bernard Lown) which was a heavily damped sinusoidal impulse having a mainly uniphasic characteristic.

Biphasic defibrillation, alternates the direction of the pulses, completing one cycle in approximately 10 milliseconds. Biphasic defibrillation was originally developed and used for implantable cardioverter-defibrillators. When applied to external defibrillators, biphasic defibrillation significantly decreases the energy level necessary for successful defibrillation, decreasing the risk of burns and myocardial damage.

Ventricular fibrillation (VF) could be returned to normal sinus rhythm in 60% of cardiac arrest patients treated with a single shock from a monophasic defibrillator. Most biphasic defibrillators have a first shock success rate of greater than 90%.

Implantable devices

A further development in defibrillation came with the invention of the implantable device, known as an implantable cardioverter- defibrillator (or ICD). This was pioneered at Sinai Hospital in Baltimore by a team that included Stephen Heilman, Alois Langer, Jack Lattuca, Morton Mower, Michel Mirowski, and Mir Imran, with the help of industrial collaborator Intec Systems of PittsburghMirowski eamed up with Mower and Staewen, and together they commenced their research in 1969 but it was 11 years before they treated their first patient. Similar developmental work was carried out by Schuder and colleagues at the University of Missouri.

The work was commenced, despite doubts amongst leading experts in the field of arrhythmias and sudden death. There was doubt that their ideas would ever become a clinical reality. In 1962 Bernard Lown introduced the external DC defibrillator. This device applied a direct current from a discharging capacitor through the chest wall into the heart to stop heart fibrillation. In 1972, Lown stated in the journal *Circulation* — "The very rare patient who has frequent bouts of ventricular fibrillation is best treated in a

coronary care unit and is better served by an effective antiarrhythmic program or surgical correction of inadequate coronary blood flow or ventricular malfunction. In fact, the implanted defibrillator system represents an imperfect solution in search of a plausible and practical application."

The problems to be overcome were the design of a system which would allow detection of ventricular fibrillation or ventricular tachycardia. Despite the lack of financial backing and grants, they persisted and the first device was implanted in February 1980 at Johns Hopkins Hospital by Dr. Levi Watkins, Jr. Modern ICDs do not require a thoracotomy and possess pacing, cardioversion, and defibrillation capabilities.

The invention of implantable units is invaluable to some regular sufferers of heart problems, although they are generally only given to those people who have already had a cardiac episode.

Types

Manual external defibrillator

The units are used in conjunction with (or more often have inbuilt) electrocardiogram readers, which the healthcare provider uses to diagnose a cardiac condition (most often fibrillation or tachycardia although there are some other rhythms which can be treated by different shocks).

The healthcare provider will then decide what charge (in joules) to use, based on proven guidelines and experience, and will deliver the shock through paddles or pads on the patient's chest. As they require detailed medical knowledge, these units are generally only found in hospitals and on some ambulances.

Manual internal defibrillator

These are the direct descendants of the work of Beck and Lown. They are virtually identical to the external version, except that the charge is delivered through internal paddles in direct contact with the heart. These are almost exclusively found in operating theatres, where the chest is likely to be open, or can be opened quickly by a surgeon.

Automated external defibrillator (AED)

These simple-to-use units are based on computer technology which is designed to analyze the heart rhythm itself, and then advise the user whether a shock is required. They are designed to be used by lay persons, who require little training to operate them correctly. They are usually limited in their interventions to delivering high joule shocks for VF (ventricular fibrillation) and VT (ventricular tachycardia) rhythms, making them generally of limited use to health professionals, who could diagnose and treat a wider range of problems with a manual or semi-automatic unit.

The automatic units also take time (generally 10–20 seconds) to diagnose the rhythm, where a professional could diagnose and treat the condition far more quickly with a manual unit These time intervals for analysis, which require stopping chest compressions, have been shown in a number of studies to have a significant negative effect on shock success This effect led to the recent change in the AHA defibrillation guideline (calling for two minutes of CPR after each shock without analyzing the cardiac rhythm) and some bodies recommend that AEDs should not be used when manual defibrillators and trained operators are available.

Automated external defibrillators are generally either held by trained personnel who will attend incidents, or are public access units which can be found in places including corporate and government offices, shopping centers, airports, restaurants, casinos, hotels, sports stadiums, schools and universities, community centers, fitness centers and

In many areas, emergency services vehicles are likely to carry AEDs. EMT-Basics in most areas are not trained in manual defibrillation, and often carry an AED instead. Some ambulances carry an AED in addition to a manual unit. In addition, some police or fire service vehicles carry an AED for first responder use. Some areas have dedicated community first responders, who are

volunteers tasked with keeping an AED and taking it to any victims in their area. It is also increasingly common to find AEDs on transport such as commercial airlines and cruise ships. The presence of an AED can be a particularly decisive factor in cardiac patient survival in these scenarios, as professional medical assistance may be hours away.

There are 2 types of AEDs: Fully Automated and Semi Automated. Most AEDs are semi-automated. A semi-automated AED automatically diagnoses heart rhythms and determines if a shock is necessary. If a shock is advised, the user must then push a button to administer the shock. A fully automated AED automatically diagnoses the heart rhythm and advises the user to stand back while the shock is automatically given. Also, some types of AEDs come with advanced features, such as a manual override or

an ECG displays.

Implantable cardioverter-defibrillator (ICD)

Also known as automatic internal cardiac defibrillator (AICD). These devices are implants, similar to pacemakers (and many can also perform the pace making function). They constantly monitor the patient's heart rhythm, and automatically administer shocks for various life-threatening arrhythmias, according to the device's programming. Many modern devices can distinguish between ventricular fibrillation, ventricular tachycardia, and more benign arrhythmias like supraventricular tachycardia and atrial fibrillation. Some devices may attempt overdrive pacing prior to synchronized cardioversion. When the life-threatening arrhythmia is ventricular fibrillation, the device is programmed to proceed immediately to an unsynchronized shock.

There are cases where the patient's ICD may fire constantly or inappropriately. This is considered a medical emergency, as it depletes the device's battery life, causes significant discomfort and anxiety to the patient, and in some cases may actually trigger life threatening arrhythmias. Some emergency medical services personnel are now equipped with a ring magnet to place over the device, which effectively disables the shock function of the device while still allowing the pacemaker to function (if the device is so equipped). If the device is shocking frequently, but appropriately, EMS personnel may administer sedation.

Wearable cardiac defibrillator

A development of the AICD is a portable external defibrillator that is worn like a vest. The unit monitors the patient 24 hours a day and will automatically deliver a biphasic shock if needed. This device is mainly indicated in patients awaiting an implantable defibrillator. Currently only one company manufactures these and they are of limited availability.

CHAPTER NINETEEN

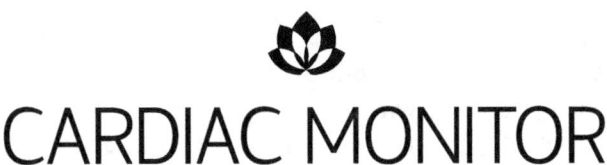

CARDIAC MONITOR

Definition

The cardiac monitor is a device that shows the heart's electrical activity as a wave pattern on a monitor. It is a bedside monitor.

Purpose

The cardiac monitor continuously shows the cardiac rhythm and sends the electrocardiogram (EKG) tracing to a main monitor in the nursing station. Most commonly used in emergency rooms and critical care areas, cardiac monitoring allows for continual observation of several patients. Aside from monitoring cardiac patients, continuous monitoring is useful for observation of postoperative patients, patients with severe electrolyte imbalances, and other unstable patients. Continuous cardiac monitoring allows for prompt identification and initiation of treatment for cardiac arrhythmias and other conditions.

Precautions

The American Heart Association warns of potential interference between some pacemakers and cardiac monitors. Minute ventilation rate-adaptive pacemakers can occasionally interact with certain cardiac monitoring and diagnostic equipment, causing the pacemakers to pace at their maximum-programmed rate. Minute ventilation is sensed in rate-adaptive pacemakers by technology known as bioelectric impedance measurement (BIM). Many medical devices in addition to pacemakers use this technology. When one of these devices is used on a patient with an active, minute ventilation rate-adaptive pacemaker, the pacemaker can erroneously interpret the mixture of BIM signals created in the patient, resulting in an elevated pacing rate. Cardiac monitors, echocardiograph equipment, apnea monitors, respiration monitors, and external defibrillators are common devices that may use BIM technology.

Description

The monitor provides a visual display of the patient's heart rhythm, which is particularly useful information during heart attacks, when patients can develop lethal cardiac arrhythmias. The monitor sounds an alarm if the patient's heart rate goes above or below a predetermined number. An automatic blood pressure cuff and a pulse oximeter, which measures the oxygen saturation in the blood, are also included with some monitors.

Equipment required for continuous cardiac monitoring includes:
cardiac monitor
monitor cable
lead wires
electrodes
dry washcloth or gauze pad
alcohol sponges

Preparation

All electrical equipment and outlets are grounded to avoid electrical shock and artifact (electrical activity caused by interference). The nurse should plug in the monitor, turn on power, and connect the cable if not already attached. He or she should connect the lead wires to the proper position and ensure that color-coded wires match the color-coded cable. If the device is not color coded, the right arm (RA) wire should be attached to the RA outlet, the left arm (LA) wire attached to the LA outlet, and so forth. The nurse should open the electrode package, and attach an electrode to each lead wire. The hands should be washed and the procedure should be explained to the patient. Privacy should be ensured for the patient, and the patient should be clean and dry to prevent electrical shock.

Next, the chest should be exposed and the sites selected for electrode placement. Using the rough patch on the electrode, a dry washcloth, or gauze pad, each site should be rubbed briskly until it reddens, but care should be taken not to damage or break the skin. Dead skin cells are removed in this manner, thereby promoting better electrical conduction. Patients who are extremely hairy may need to be shaved prior to application of the electrodes. An alcohol pad is used to clean the sites in patients with oily skin. Areas should dry completely to promote good adhesion. Alcohol should not become trapped beneath the electrode, as this can lead to skin breakdown. In addition to oily skin, diaphoretic skin can cause interference in the recording. To minimize this interference, the electrode site should be rubbed with a dry 4x4 gauze pad before application. The backing of the electrode should be removed, and the gel inspected. If the electrode has dried out, which can happen if the electrode package is opened before immediate use, it should be discarded and another used. The nurse should apply one electrode to each site, press one side of the electrode against the skin, and pull gently. Then, the opposite side of the electrode should be pressed against the skin. The nurse should press two fingers on the electrode in a circular pattern to affix the gel and stabilize the electrode, then repeat for each electrode. *To avoid potential artifact, do not place the electrodes on bony prominences or hairy areas.*

Aftercare

After placing all electrodes, the nurse should observe the monitor and evaluate the quality of the tracing, make ing size and tracing position adjustments as needed. He or she should confirm that the monitor is detecting each heartbeat by taking an apical pulse and comparing the pulse to the digital display. The upper and lower alarm limits should be set according to institutional policy, and the alarm activated. A rhythm strip should be recorded for the medical record, and labeled with patient name, room number, date, time, and interpretation of the strip.

Complications

There is a potential for skin breakdown at the electrode placement site. The patient may be allergic to the adhesive used, or the electrode may have been left on the skin too long. The electrodes should be removed and new electrodes applied, using hypoallergenic electrodes if necessary.

Results

A normal cardiac tracing shows a regular rate and rhythm with no deviations in the QRST complex (the combined waves of an electrocardiogram). Abnormal results may include bradycardia, or tachycardia, accompanied by the alarm. Q waves (the short initial downward stroke of the QRST complex) are abnormal, and may or may not signal an infarction.

Some causes of noninfarction Q waves are:
ventricular hypertrophy
ventricular preexcitation (Wolf-Parkinson-White syndrome)

cardiomyopathies
pulmonary embolism
incomplete left bundle branch block

Causes of changes in ST Segment (part of the EKG between the QRS complex and the T wave) and T Wave (deflection in an EKG that represents electrical activity of the ventricular repolarization) include:

aberrant conduction
amyloidosis
bundle branch block
cardiomyopathy
cocaine vasospasm
electrolyte disturbances
intracranial hemorrhage
myocardial metastases
myocarditis
paced rhythm
pancreatitis or acute abdomen
pericarditis
physical training
Printzmetal's angina
pulmonary embolism
tachycardia
ventricular aneurysm
ventricular hypertrophy
ventricular rhythms
Wolff-Parkinson-White syndrome

Alarm signals are abnormal and must be investigated. A false high alarm rate may be caused by skeletal muscle activity or by the monitor incorrectly interpreting large T waves as a QRS complex, which would double the true heart rate. The electrodes should be repositioned as needed to ensure that the electrode is not over a major muscle mass and that QRS complex is larger than the T wave. A false low alarm rate may be due to patient movement, or poor contact between electrodes and skin. Electrodes should be reapplied as needed. Artifact is a common abnormal finding, and may be caused by improperly placed electrodes, patient movement, static electricity, seizures, anxiety, or chills. The position of electrodes should be checked and static-causing bed linen changed. The cables should not have exposed connectors.

CHAPTER TWENTY

HEMIPLEGIA & PARAPLEGIA

Hemiplegia

Hemiplegia is total paralysis of the arm, leg, and trunk on the same side of the body. Hemiplegia is more severe than hemiparesis, wherein one half of the body has less marked weakness Hemiplegia may be congenital or acquired from an illness or stroke.

Hemiplegia is not an uncommon medical disorder. In elderly individuals, strokes are the most common cause of hemiplegia. In children, the majority of cases of hemiplegia have no identifiable cause and occur with a frequency of about one in every thousand births. Experts indicate that the majority of case es of hemiplegia that occur up to the age of two should be considered to be cerebral palsy until proven otherwise.

Causes

The most common cause of hemiplegia is a cerebrovascular accident, also known as a stroke. Strokes can cause a variety of movement disorders, depending on the location and severity of the lesion. Hemiplegia is common when the stroke affects the corticospinal tract. Other causes of hemiplegia include spinal cord injury, specifically Brown-Sequard syndrome, traumatic brain injury, or disease affecting the brain. As a lesion that results in hemiplegia occurs in the brain or spinal cord, hemiplegic muscles display features of the Upper Motor Neuron Syndrome. Features other than weakness include decreased movement control, clonus (a series of involuntary rapid muscle contractions), spasticity, exaggerated deep tendon reflexes and decreased endurance.

It is well known that the incidence of hemiplegia is a lot higher in premature babies than term babies. There is also a high incidence of hemiplegia during pregnancy and experts believe that this may be related to either a traumatic delivery, use of forceps or some event which causes brain injury.

Hemiplegia in adults include trauma, bleeding, brain infections and cancers. Individuals who have uncontrolled diabetes, hypertension or those who smoke have a higher chance of developing a stroke. Weakness on one side of the face may occur and may be due to a viral infection, stroke or a cancer.

Medial medullary syndrome Common causes by etiology

Vascular: cerebral hemorrhage, stroke, diabetic neuropathy

Infective: encephalitis, meningitis, brain abscess

Neoplastic: glioma-meningioma

Demyelination: disseminated sclerosis, lesions to the internal capsule

     Traumatic: cerebral lacerations, subdural hematoma rare cause of hemiplegia is due to local an aesthetic injection given intra-arterially rapidly, instead of given in a nerve branch.

Congenital: cerebral palsy

Disseminated: multiple sclerosis

Psychological: parasomnia (nocturnal hemiplegia) [Pathogenesis

The exact cause of hemiplegia is not known in all cases, but it appears that the brain is deprived of oxygen and this results in the death of neurons. When the corticospinal tract is damaged, the injury is usually manifested on the opposite side of the body. For example, if one has an injury to the right side of the brain, the hemiplegia will be on the left side of the body.

Signs and Symptoms

Hemiplegia means severe weakness of the limbs on one side of the body but the specific features can vary tremendously from person to person. Problems may include:
- Difficulty with gait
- Difficulty with balance while standing or walking
- Having difficulty with motor activities like holding, grasping or pinching
- Increasing stiffness of muscles
- Muscle spasms
- Difficulty with speech
- Difficulty swallowing food
- Significant delay in achieving developmental milestones like standing, smiling, crawling or speaking The majority of children who develop hemiplegia also have abnormal mental development Behavior problems like anxiety, anger, irritability, lack of concentration or comprehension
- Emotions- depression

Diagnosis

Hemiplegia is identified by clinical examination by a health professional, such as a physiotherapist or doctor. Radiological studies like a CT scan or magnetic resonance imaging of the brain should be used to
confirm injury in the brain and spinal cord, but alone cannot be used to identify movement disorders. Individuals who develop seizures may undergo tests to determine where the focus of excess electrical activity is.

Hemiplegia patients usually show a characteristic gait. The leg on the affected side is extended and internally rotated and is swung in a wide, lateral arc rather than lifted in order to move it forward. The upper limb on the same side is also adducted at the shoulder, flexed at the elbow, and pronated at the wrist with the thumb tucked into the palm and the fingers curled around it.

Treatment

Treatment should be based on assessment by the relevant health professionals, including physiotherapists, doctors and occupational therapists. Muscles with severe motor impairment including weakness need these therapists to assist them with specific exercise, and are likely to require help to do this.

Drugs can be used to treat issues related to the Upper Motor Neuron Syndrome. Drugs like Librium or Valium could be used as a relaxant. Drugs are also given to individuals whom have recurrent seizures, which may be a separate but related problem after brain injury.

Surgery may be used if the individual develops a secondary issue of contracture, from a severe imbalance of muscle activity. In such cases the surgeon may cut the ligaments and relieve joint contractures. Individuals who are unable to swallow may have a tube inserted into the stomach. This allows food to be given directly into the stomach. The food is in liquid form and instilled at low rates. Prosthetics. Some individuals with hemiplegia will benefit from some type of prosthetic device. There are many types of braces and splints available to stabilize a joint, assist with walking and keep the upper body erect.

Rehabilitation is the main treatment of individuals with hemiplegia. In all cases, the major aim of rehabilitation is to regain maximum function and quality of life. Both physical and occupational therapy can significantly improve the quality of life. Physical therapy can help improve muscle strength, mobility such as standing and walking, and other physical function. Occupational therapy may help the individual train daily living activities like brushing teeth, combing hair or dressing. Initially, one may undergo physical therapy at a center but many of these exercises can also be done at home and become part of daily life routine. A treatment method that can be implement with the goal of helping to regain motor function in the affected limb is constraint-induced movement therapy. Treatments consist of constraining the unaffected limb, forcing the affected limb to accomplish tasks of daily living.

There are a variety of standardized assessment scales available to physiotherapists and other health care professionals for use in the ongoing evaluation of the status of a patient's hemiplegia. The use of standardized assessment scales may help physiotherapists and other health care professionals during the course of their treatment plant to:

Prioritize treatment interventions based on specific identifiable motor and sensory deficits

Create appropriate short- and long-term goals for treatment based on the outcome of the scales, their professional expertise and the desires of the patient

Evaluate the potential burden of care and monitor any changes based on either improving or declining scores Three of the most commonly used scales in the assessment of hemiplegia are:

The Fugl-Meyer Assessment of Physical Performance (FMA)-The FMA is often used as a measure of functional or physical impairment following a cerebrovascular accident (CVA). It measures sensory and motor impairment of the upper and lower extremities, balance in several positions, range of motion, and pain. This test is a reliable and valid measure in measuring post-stroke impairments related to stroke recovery. A lower score in each component of the test indicates higher impairment and a lower functional level for that area. The maximum score for each component is 66 for the upper extremities, 34 for the lower extremities, and 14 for balance.

The Chedoke-McMaster Stroke Assessment (CMSA)

-This test is a reliable measure of two separate components evaluating both motor impairment and disability the disability component assesses any changes in physical function including gross motor function and walking ability. The disability inventory can have a maximum score of 100 with 70 from the gross motor index and 30 from the walking index. Each task in this inventory has a maximum score of seven except for the 2-minute walk test which is out of two. The impairment component of the test evaluates the upper and lower extremities, postural control and pain. The impairment inventory focuses on the seven stages of recovery from stroke from flaccid paralysis to normal motor functioning.

The Stroke Rehabilitation Assessment of Movement (STREAM) The STREAM consists of 30 test items involving upper-limb movements, lower-limb movements, and basic mobility items. It is a clinical measure of voluntary movements and general mobility (rolling, bridging, sit-to-stand, standing, stepping, walking and stairs) following a stroke. The voluntary movement part of the assessment is measured using a 3-point ordinal scale (unable to perform, partial performance, and complete performance) and the mobility part of the assessment uses a 4-point ordinal scale (unable, partial, complete with aid, complete no aid). The maximum score one can receive on the STREAM is a 70 (20 for each limb score and 30 for mobility score). The higher the score, the better movement and mobility is available for the individual being scored.

Prognosis

Hemiplegia is not a progressive disorder, except in progressive conditions like a growing brain tumor. Once the injury has occurred, the symptoms should not worsen. However, because of lack of mobility, other complications can occur. Complications may include muscle and joint stiffness, loss of aerobic fitness, muscle spasms, bed sores, pressure ulcers and blood clots. Sudden recovery from hemiplegia is very rare. Many of the individuals will have limited recovery, but the majority will improve from intensive, specialized rehabilitation. Potential to progress may differ in cerebral palsy, compared to adult acquired brain injury. It is vital to integrate the hemiplegic child into society and encourage them in their daily living activities. With time, some individuals may make remarkable progress.

Paraplegia

Paraplegia is an impairment in motor or sensory function of the lower extremities. The word comes from Ionic Greek: "half-striking". It is usually the result of spinal cord injuryor a congenital condition such as spina bifida which affects the neural elements of the spinal canal. The area of the spinal canal which is affected in paraplegia is either the thoracic, lumbar, or sacral regions. If both arms are also affected by paralysis, quadriplegia is the proper terminology. If only one limb is affected the correct term is monoplegia.

Spastic paraplegia is a form of paraplegia defined by spasticity of the affected muscles, rather than flaccid paralysis.

While some people with paraplegia can walk to a degree, many are dependent on wheelchairs or other supportive measures. Depending on the level and extent of spinal damage, people with paraplegia may experience some, or complete loss of sensation in the affected limbs. Impotence and various degreesof urinary and fecal incontinence may also occur. Many use catheters or a bowel management program (often involving suppositories, enemas, or digital stimulation of the bowels) to address these problems. With successful bladder and bowel management, paraplegics can prevent virtually all accidental urinary or bowel discharges. Some paraplegics prefer the use of incontinence products such as Depend as an alternative.

Complications

Due to the decrease or loss of feeling or function in the lower extremities, paraplegia can contribute to a number of medical complications to include pressure sores (decubitus), thrombosis and pneumonia. Physiotherapy and various assistive technology, such as a standing frame, as well as vigilant self-observation and care may aid in helping to prevent future and mitigate existing complications.

As paraplegia is most often the result of a traumatic injury to the spinal cord tissue and the resulting inflammation, other nerve related complications can and do occur. Cases of chronic nerve pain in the areas surrounding the point of injury are not uncommon. There is speculation that the "phantom pains" experienced by individuals suffering from paralysis could be a direct result of these collateral nerve injuries misinterpreted by the brain

CHAPTER TWENTY-ONE

PARALYSIS & PARKINSON DISEASE

Paralysis

Paralysis is loss of muscle function for one or more muscles. Paralysis can be accompanied by a loss of feeling (sensory loss) in the affected area if there is sensory damage as well as motor. A study conducted by the Christopher & Dana Reeve Foundation, suggests that about 1 in 50 people have been diagnosed with paralysis. The word comes from the Greek means "disabling of the nerves".

Causes

Paralysis is most often caused by damage in the nervous system, especially the spinal cord. Other major causes are stroke, trauma with nerve injury, poliomyelitis, amyotrophic lateral sclerosis (ALS), botulism, spina bifida, multiple sclerosis, and Guillain-Barré syndrome. Temporary paralysis occurs during REM sleep, and dysregulation of this system can lead to episodes of waking paralysis. Drugs that interfere with nerve function, such as curare, can also cause paralysis. There are many known causes for paralysis, and perhaps more yet to be discovered.

Pseudo paralysis (*pseudo-* meaning "false, not genuine", from Greek ψεῦδος) is voluntary restriction or inhibition of motion because of pain, incoordination, or other cause, and is not due to actual muscular paralysis in an infant, it may be a symptom of congenital syphilis.

Variations

Paralysis could be localized, or generalized, or it may follow a certain pattern. Most paralyses caused by nervous system damage (i.e. spinal cord injuries) are constant in nature; however, there are forms of periodic paralysis, including sleep paralysis, which are caused by other factors.

Parkinson's disease

a degenerative disorder of the central nervous system. It results from the death of dopamine-containing cells in thesubstantia nigra, a region of the midbrain; the cause of cell-death is unknown. Early in the course of the disease, the most obvious symptoms are movement-related, including shaking, rigidity, slowness of movement and difficulty with walking and gait. Later, cognitive and behavioral problems may arise, with dementia commonly occurring in the advanced stages of the disease. Other symptoms include sensory, sleep and emotional problems. PD is more common in the elderly with most cases occurring after the age of 50.

The main motor symptoms are collectively called parkinsonism, or a "parkinsonian syndrome". Parkinson's disease is often defined as a parkinsonian syndrome that is idiopathic (having no known cause), although some atypical cases have a genetic origin. Many risk and protective factors have been investigated: the clearest evidence is for an increased risk of PD in people exposed to certain pesticides and a reduced risk in tobacco smokers. The pathology of the disease is characterized by the accumulation of a protein called alpha-synuclein into inclusions called Lewy bodies in neurons, and from insufficient formation and activity of dopamine produced in certain neurons of parts of the midbrain.

Diagnosis of typical cases is mainly based on symptoms, with tests such as neuroimaging being used for confirmation.

Modern treatments are effective at managing the early motor symptoms of the disease, mainly through the use of levodopa and dopamine agonists. As the disease progresses and dopamine neurons continue to be lost, a point eventually arrives at which these drugs become ineffective at treating the symptoms and at the same time produce a complication called dyskinesia, marked by involuntary writhing movements. Diet and some forms of rehabilitation have shown some effectiveness at alleviating symptoms. Surgery and deep brain stimulation have been used to reduce motor symptoms as a last resort in severe cases where drugs are ineffective. Research directions include a search of new animal models of the disease and investigations of the potential usefulness of gene therapy, stem cell transplants and neuroprotective agents. Medications to treat non-movement-related symptoms of PD, such as sleep disturbances and emotional problems, also exist.

The disease is named after the English doctor James Parkinson, who published the first detailed description in *An Essay on the Shaking Palsy* in 1817. Several major organizations promote research and improvement of quality of life of those with the disease and their families. Public awareness campaigns include Parkinson's disease day on the birthday of James Parkinson, April 11, and the use of a red tulip as the symbol of the disease. People with parkinsonism who have enhanced the public's awareness include Michael J.

Classification

The term parkinsonism is used for a motor syndrome whose main symptoms are tremor at rest, stiffness, slowing of movement and postural instability. Parkinsonian syndromes can be divided into four subtypes according to their origin: primary or idiopathic, secondary or acquired, hereditary parkinsonism, and Parkinson plus syndromes or multiple system degeneration. Parkinson's disease is the most common form of parkinsonism and is usually defined as "primary" parkinsonism, meaning parkinsonism with no external identifiable cause. In recent years several genes that are directly related to some cases of Parkinson's disease have been discovered. As much as this can go against the definition of Parkinson's disease as an idiopathic illness, genetic parkinsonism disorders with a similar clinical course to PD are generally included under the Parkinson's disease label. The terms "familial Parkinson's disease" and "sporadic Parkinson's disease" can be used to differentiate genetic from truly idiopathic forms of the disease.

PD is usually classified as a movement disorder, although it also gives rise to several non- motor types of symptoms such as sensory deficits, cognitive difficulties or sleep problems. Parkinson plus diseases are primary parkinsonism's which present additional features. They include multiple system atrophy, progressive supranuclear palsy, corticobasal degeneration and dementia with Lewy bodies.

In terms of pathophysiology, PD is considered a synucleinopathy due to an abnormal accumulation of alpha-synuclein protein in the brain in the form of Lewy bodies, as opposed to other diseases such as Alzheimer's disease where the brain accumulates tau protein in the form of neurofibrillary tangles. Nevertheless, there is clinical and pathological overlap between tauopathies and synucleinopathies. The most typical symptom of Alzheimer's disease, dementia, occurs in advanced stages of PD, while it is common to find neurofibrillary tangles in brains affected by PD.

Dementia with Lewy bodies (DLB) is another synucleinopathy that has similarities with PD, and especially with the subset of PD cases with dementia. However, the relationship between PD and DLB is complex and still has to be clarified. They may represent parts of a continuum or they may be separate diseases.

Signs and symptoms

Parkinson's disease affects movement, producing motor symptoms.Non-motor symptoms, which include autonomic dysfunction, neuropsychiatric problems (mood, cognition, behavior or thought alterations), and sensory and sleep difficulties, are also common.

Motor

Four motor symptoms are considered cardinal in PD: tremor, rigidity, slowness of movement, and postural instability.

Tremor is the most apparent and well-known symptom. It is the most common; though around 30% of individuals with PD do not have tremor at disease onset, most develop it as the disease progresses. It is usually a rest tremor: maximal when the limb is at rest and disappearing with voluntary movement and sleep. It affects to a greater extent the most distal part of the limb and at onset typically appears in only a single arm or leg, becoming bilateral later. Frequency of PD tremor is between 4 and 6 hertz (cycles per second). A feature of tremor is "pill-rolling", a term used to describe the tendency of the index finger of the hand to get into contact with the thumb and perform together a circular movement. The term derives from the similarity between the movement in PD patients and the earlier pharmaceutical technique of manually making pills.

Bradykinesia (slowness of movement) is another characteristic feature of PD, and is associated with difficulties along the whole course of the movement process, from planning to initiation and finally execution of a movement. Performance of sequential and simultaneous movement is hindered. Bradykinesia is the most disabling symptom in the early stages of the disease. Initial manifestations are problems when performing daily tasks which require fine motor control such as writing, sewing or getting dressed. Clinical evaluation is based in similar tasks such as alternating movements between both hands or both feet. Bradykinesia is not equal for all movements or times. It is modified by the activity or emotional state of the subject, to the point that some patients are barely able to walk yet can still ride a bicycle. Generally, patients have less difficulty when some sort of external cue is provided.

Rigidity is stiffness and resistance to limb movement caused by increased muscle tone, an excessive and continuous contraction of muscles. In parkinsonism the rigidity can be uniform (lead-pipe rigidity) or ratchet (cogwheel rigidity). The combination of tremor and increased tone is considered to be at the origin of cogwheel rigidity. Rigidity may be associated with joint pain; such pain being a frequent initial manifestation of the disease.

In early stages of Parkinson's disease, rigidity is often asymmetrical and it tends to affect the neck and shoulder muscles prior to the muscles of the face and extremities. With the progression of the disease, rigidity typically affects the whole body and reduces the ability to move.

Postural instability is typical in the late stages of the disease, leading to impaired balance and frequent falls, and secondarily to bone fractures. Instability is often absent in the initial stages, especially in younger people. Up to 40% of the patients may experience falls and around 10% may have falls weekly, with number of falls being related to the severity of PD.

Other recognized motor signs and symptoms include gait and posture disturbances such as festination (rapid shuffling steps and a forward-flexed posture when walking), speech and swallowing disturbances including voice disorders, mask-like face expression or small handwriting, although the range of possible motor problems that can appear is large.

Neuropsychiatric

Parkinson's disease can cause neuropsychiatric disturbances which can range from mild to severe. This includes disorders of cognition, mood, behavior, and thought. Cognitive disturbances can occur in the initial stages of the disease and sometimes prior to diagnosis, and increase in prevalence with duration of the disease. The most common cognitive deficit in affected individuals is executive dysfunction, which can include problems with planning, cognitive flexibility, abstract thinking, rule acquisition, initiating appropriate actions and inhibiting inappropriate actions, and selecting relevant sensory information. Fluctuations in attention and slowed cognitive speed are among other cognitive difficulties. Memory is affected, specifically in recalling learned information. Nevertheless, improvement appears when recall is aided by cues. Visuospatial difficulties are also part of the disease, seen for example when the individual is asked to perform tests of facial recognition and perception of the orientation of drawn lines. A person with PD has two to six times the risk of suffering dementia compared to the general population. The prevalence of dementia increases with duration of the disease. Dementia is associated with a reduced quality of life in people with PD and their caregivers, increased mortality, and a higher probability of needing nursing home care.

Behavior and mood alterations are more common in PD without cognitive impairment than in the general population, and are usually present in PD with dementia. The most frequent mood difficulties are depression, apathy and anxiety. Impulse control behaviors such as medication overuse and craving, binge eating, hypersexuality, or pathological gambling can appear in PD and have been related to the medications used to manage the disease. Psychotic symptoms—hallucinations or delusions—occur in 4% of patients, and it is assumed that the main precipitant of psychotic phenomena in Parkinson's disease is dopaminergic excess secondary to treatment; it therefore becomes more common with increasing age and levodopa intake.

Other

In addition to cognitive and motor symptoms, PD can impair other body functions. Sleep problems are a feature of the disease and can be worsened by medications. Symptoms can manifest in daytime drowsiness, disturbances in REM sleep, or insomnia. Alterations in the autonomic nervous system can lead to orthostatic hypotension (low blood pressure upon standing), oily skin and excessive sweating, urinary incontinence and altered sexual function. Constipation and gastric dysmotility can be severe enough to cause discomfort and even endanger health. PD is related to several eye and vision abnormalities such as decreased blink rate, dry eyes, deficient ocular pursuit (eye tracking) and saccadic movements (fast automatic movements of both eyes in the same direction), difficulties in directing gaze upward, and blurred or double vision. Changes in perception may include an impaired sense of smell, sensation of pain and paresthesia (skin tingling and numbness). All of these symptoms can occur years before diagnosis of the disease.

Causes

Most people with Parkinson's disease have idiopathic Parkinson's disease (having no specific known cause). A small proportion of cases, however, can be attributed to known genetic factors. Other factors have been associated with the risk of developing PD, but no causal relationship has been proven.

PD traditionally has been considered a non-genetic disorder; however, around 15% of individuals with PD have a first-degree relative who has the disease.[2] At least 5% of people are now known to have forms of the disease that occur because of a mutation of one of several specific genes.

Mutations in specific genes have been conclusively shown to cause PD. These genes code for alpha-synuclein (SNCA), ubiquitin carboxy-terminal hydrolase L1 (UCH-L1), parkin (PRKN), leucine-rich repeat kinase 2 (LRRK2 or dardarin), PTEN-induced putative kinase 1 (PINK1), DJ-1 and ATP13A2. In most cases, people with these mutations will develop PD. With the exception of LRRK2, however, they account for only a small minority of cases of PD the most extensively studied PD-related genes are SNCA and LRRK2. Mutations in genes including SNCA, LRRK2 and glucocerebrosidase (GBA) have been found to be risk factors for sporadic PD. Mutations in GBA are known to cause Gaucher's disease. Genome-wide association studies, which search for mutated alleles with low penetrance in sporadic cases, have yielded few positive results, but such studies have been few in number and their size small.

The role of the SNCA gene is important in PD because the alpha-synuclein protein is the main component of Lewy bodies. Missense mutations of the gene (in which a single nucleotide is changed), and duplications and triplications of the locus containing it have been found in different groups with familial PD. Missense mutations are rare. On the other hand, multiplications of the SNCA locus account for around 2% of familial cases. Multiplications have been found in asymptomatic carriers, which indicate that penetrance is incomplete or age-dependent.

The LRRK2 gene (PARK8) encodes for a protein called dardarin. The name dardarin was taken from a Basque word for tremor, because this gene was first identified in families from England and the north of Spain.

Mutations in LRRK2 are the most commonly known cause of familial and sporadic PD, accounting for up to 10% of individuals with a family history of the disease and 3% of sporadic cases. More than 40 different mutations of the gene have been found to be related to PD.

Pathology

Anatomical pathology

The basal ganglia, a group of "brain structures" innervated by the dopaminergic system, are the most seriously affected brain areas in PD. The main pathological characteristic of PD is cell death in the substantia nigra and, more specifically, the ventral (front) part of the pars compacta, affecting up to 70% of the cells by the time death occurs.

Macroscopic alterations can be noticed on cut surfaces of the brainstem, where neuronal loss can be inferred from a reduction of melanin pigmentation in the substantia nigra and locus coeruleus. The histopathology (microscopic anatomy) of the substantia nigra and several other brain regions shows neuronal loss and Lewy bodies in many of the remaining nerve cells. Neuronal loss is accompanied by death of astrocytes (star-shaped glial cells) and activation of the microglia (another type of glial cell). Lewy bodies are a key pathological feature of PD.

Pathophysiology

The primary symptoms of Parkinson's disease result from greatly reduced activity of dopamine-secreting cells caused by cell death in the pars compacta region of the substantia nigra. There are five major pathways in the brain connecting other brain areas with the basal ganglia. These are known as the motor, oculomotor, associative, limbic and orbitofrontal circuits, with names indicating the main projection area of each circuit. All of them are affected in PD, and their disruption explains many of the symptoms of the disease since these circuits are involved in a wide variety of functions including movement, attention and learning. Scientifically, the motor circuit has been examined the most intensively.

A particular conceptual model of the motor circuit and its alteration with PD has been of great influence since 1980, although some limitations have been pointed out which have led to modifications. In this model, the basal ganglia normally exert a constant inhibitory influence on a wide range of motor systems, preventing them from becoming active at inappropriate times. When a decision is made to perform a particular action, inhibition is reduced for the required motor system, thereby releasing it for activation. Dopamine acts to facilitate this release of inhibition, so high levels of dopamine function tend to promote motor activity, while low levels of dopamine function, such as occur in PD, demand greater exertions of effort for any given movement. Thus, the net effect of dopamine depletion is to produce hypokinesia, an overall reduction in motor output. Drugs that are used to treat PD, conversely, may produce excessive dopamine activity, allowing motor systems to be activated at inappropriate times and thereby producing dyskinesias.

Brain cell death

There is speculation of several mechanisms by which the brain cells could be lost. One mechanism consists of an abnormal accumulation of the protein alpha-synuclein bound to ubiquitin in the damaged cells. This insoluble protein accumulates inside neurons forming inclusions called Lewy bodies. According to the Braak staging, a classification of the disease based on pathological findings, Lewy bodies first appear in the olfactory bulb, medulla oblongata and pontine tegmentum, with individuals at this stage being asymptomatic. As the disease progresses, Lewy bodies later develop in the substantia nigra, areas of the midbrain and basal forebrain, and in a last step the neocortex. These brain sites are the main places of neuronal degeneration in PD; however, Lewy bodies may not cause cell death and they may be protective. In patients with dementia, a generalized presence of Lewy bodies is common in cortical areas. Neurofibrillary tangles and senile plaques, characteristic of Alzheimer's disease, are not common unless the person is demented.

Other cell-death mechanisms include proteasomal and lysosomal system dysfunction and reduced mitochondrial activity. Iron accumulation in the substantia nigra is typically observed in conjunction with the protein inclusions. It may be related to oxidative stress, protein aggregation and neuronal death, but the mechanisms are not fully understood.

Diagnosis

A physician will diagnose Parkinson's disease from the medical history and a neurological examination. There is no lab test that will clearly identify the disease, but brain scans are sometimes used to rule out disorders that could give rise to similar symptoms. Patients may be given levodopa and resulting relief of motor impairment tends to confirm diagnosis. The finding of Lewy bodies in the midbrain on autopsy is usually considered proof that the patient suffered from Parkinson's disease. The progress of the illness over time may reveal it is not Parkinson's disease, and some authorities recommend that the diagnosis be periodically reviewed.

Other causes that can secondarily produce a parkinsonian syndrome are Alzheimer's disease, multiple cerebral infarction and drug-induced parkinsonism. Parkinson plus syndromes such as progressive supranuclear palsy and multiple system atrophy must be ruled out.[1] Anti-Parkinson's medications are typically less effective at controlling symptoms in Parkinson plus syndromes. Faster progression rates, early cognitive dysfunction or postural instability, minimal tremor or symmetry at onset may indicate a Parkinson plus disease rather than PD itself. Genetic forms are usually classified as PD, although the terms *familial Parkinson's disease* and *familial parkinsonism* are used for disease entities with an autosomal dominant or recessive pattern of inheritance.

Medical organizations have created diagnostic criteria to ease and standardize the diagnostic process, especially in the early stages of the disease. The most widely known criteria come from the Parkinson's Disease Society Brain Bank and the US National Institute of Neurological Disorders and Stroke. The PD Society Brain Bank criteria require slowness of movement (bradykinesia) plus either rigidity, resting tremor, or postural instability. Other possible causes for these symptoms need to be ruled out. Finally, three or more of the following features are required during onset or evolution: unilateral onset, tremor at rest, progression in time, asymmetry of motor symptoms, response to levodopa for at least five years, clinical course of at least ten years and appearance of dyskinesias induced by the intake of excessive levodopa. Accuracy of diagnostic criteria evaluated at autopsy is 75–90%, with specialists such as neurologists having the highest rates.

Computed tomography (CT) and magnetic resonance imaging (MRI) brain scans of people with PD usually appear normal. These techniques are nevertheless useful to rule out other diseases that can be secondary causes of parkinsonism, such as basal ganglia tumors, vascular pathology and hydrocephalus. A specific technique of MRI, diffusion MRI, has been reported to be useful at discriminating between typical and atypical parkinsonism, although its exact diagnostic value is still under investigation. Dopaminergic function in the basal ganglia can be measured with different PET and SPECT radiotracers. Examples are isoflurane (trade name *DaTSCAN*) aminoketone (*Dopa scan*) for SPECT or fludeoxyglucose for PET. A pattern of reduced dopaminergic activity in the basal ganglia can aid in diagnosing PD.

Management

There is no cure for Parkinson's disease, but medications, surgery and multidisciplinary management can provide relief from the symptoms. The main families of drugs useful for treating motor symptoms are levodopa (usually combined with a dopa decarboxylase inhibitor or COMT inhibitor), dopamine agonists and MAO-B inhibitors. The stage of the disease determines which group is most useful. Two stages are usually distinguished: an initial stage in which the individual with PD has already developed some disability for which he needs pharmacological treatment, then a second stage in which an individual develops motor complications related to levodopa usage. Treatment in the initial stage aims for an optimal tradeoff between good symptom control and side-effects resulting from enhancement of dopaminergic function. The start of levodopa (or L-DOPA) treatment may be delayed by using other medications such as MAO-B inhibitors and dopamine agonists, in the hope of delaying the onset of dyskinesias. In the second stage the aim is to reduce symptoms while controlling fluctuations of the response to medication. Sudden withdrawals from medication or overuse have to be managed. When medications are not enough to control symptoms, surgery and deep brain stimulation can be of use. In the final stages of the disease, palliative care is provided to enhance quality of life.

Levodopa

Levodopa has been the most widely used treatment for over 30 years. L-DOPA is converted into dopamine in the dopaminergic neurons by dopa decarboxylase. Since motor symptoms are produced by a lack of dopamine in the substantia nigra, the administration of L-DOPA temporarily diminishes the motor symptoms.

Only 5–10% of L-DOPA crosses the blood-brain barrier. The remainder is often metabolized to dopamine elsewhere, causing a variety of side effects including nausea, dyskinesias and joint stiffness. Carbidopa and benderizine are peripheral dopa decarboxylase inhibitors, which help to prevent the metabolism of L-DOPA before it reaches the dopaminergic neurons, therefore reducing side effects and increasing bioavailability. They are generally given as combination preparations with levodopa. Existing preparations are carbidopa/levodopa (co-care dopa) and benderizine/levodopa (co-beneldopa). Levodopa has been related to dopamine dysregulation syndrome, which is a compulsive overuse of the medication, and punding. There are controlled-release versions of levodopa in the form intravenous and intestinal infusions that spread out the effect of the medication. These slow-release levodopa preparations have not shown an increased control of motor symptoms or motor complications when compared to immediate release preparations. Tolcapone inhibits the COMT enzyme, which degrades dopamine, thereby prolonging the effects of levodopa. It has been used to complement levodopa; however, its usefulness is limited by possible side effects such as liver damage. A similarly effective drug, entacapone, has not been shown to cause significant alterations of liver function. Licensed preparations of entacapone contain entacapone alone or in combination with carbidopa and levodopa.

Levodopa preparations lead in the long term to the development of motor complications characterized by involuntary movements called dyskinesias and fluctuations in the response to medication. When this occurs a person with PD can change from phases with good response to medication and few symptoms ("on" state), to phases with no response to medication and significant motor symptoms ("off" state). For this reason, levodopa doses are kept as low as possible while maintaining functionality. Delaying the initiation of therapy with levodopa by using alternatives (dopamine agonists and MAO-B inhibitors) is common practice. A former strategy to reduce motor complications was to withdraw L-DOPA medication for some time. This is discouraged now, since it can bring dangerous side effects such as neuroleptic malignant syndrome. Most people with PD will eventually need levodopa and later develop motor side effects.

Dopamine agonists

Several dopamine agonists that bind to dopaminergic post-synaptic receptors in the brain have similar effects to levodopa. These were initially used for individuals experiencing on-off fluctuations and dyskinesias as a complementary therapy to levodopa; they are now mainly used on their own as an initial therapy for motor symptoms with the aim of delaying motor complications. When used in late PD they are useful at reducing the off periods. Dopamine agonists include bromocriptine, pergolide, pramipexole, ropinirole, piribedil, cabergoline, apomorphine and lisuride.

Dopamine agonists produce significant, although usually mild, side effects including drowsiness, hallucinations, insomnia, nausea and constipation. Sometimes side effects appear even at a minimal clinically effective dose, leading the physician to search for a different drug. Compared with levodopa, dopamine agonists may delay motor complications of medication use but are less effective at controlling

symptoms. Nevertheless, they are usually effective enough to manage symptoms in the initial years. They tend to be more expensive than levodopa. Dyskinesias due to dopamine agonists are rare in younger people who have

PD, but along with other side effects, become more common with age at onset. Thus, dopamine agonists are the preferred initial treatment for earlier onset, as opposed to levodopa in later onset Agonists have been related to an impulse control disorders (such as compulsive sexual activity and eating, and pathological gambling and shopping) even more strongly than levodopa.

Apomorphine, a non-orally administered dopamine agonist, may be used to reduce off periods and dyskinesia in late PD. It is administered by intermittent injections or continuous subcutaneous infusions. Since secondary effects such as confusion and hallucinations are common, individuals receiving apomorphine treatment should be closely monitored. Two dopamine agonists that are administered through skin patches (lisuride and rotigotine) have been recently found to be useful for patients in initial stages and preliminary positive results has been published on the control of off states in patients in the advanced state.

MAO-B inhibitors

MAO-B inhibitors (selegiline and rasagiline) increase the level of dopamine in the basal ganglia by blocking its metabolism. They inhibit monoamine oxidase-B (MAO-B) which breaks down dopamine secreted by the dopaminergic neurons. The reduction in MAO-B activity results in increased L-DOPA in the striatum. Like dopamine agonists, MAO-B inhibitors used as monotherapy improve motor symptoms and delay the need for levodopa in early disease, but produce more adverse effects and are less effective than levodopa.

There are few studies of their effectiveness in the advanced stage, although results suggest that they are useful to reduce fluctuations between on and off periods. An initial study indicated that selegiline in combination with levodopa increased the risk of death, but this was later disproven.

Other drugs

Other drugs such as amantadine and anticholinergics may be useful as treatment of motor symptoms. However, the evidence supporting them lacks quality, so they are not first choice treatments. In addition to motor symptoms, PD is accompanied by a diverse range of symptoms. A number of drugs have been used to treat some of these problems. Examples are the use of clozapine for psychosis, cholinesterase inhibitors for dementia,and modafinil for daytime sleepiness.

CHAPTER TWENTY-TWO

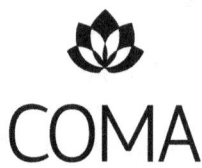

COMA

Coma

In medicine, a coma meaning deep sleep is a state of unconsciousness, lasting more than 6 hours in which a person cannot be awakened, fails to respond normally too painful stimuli, light or sound, lacks a normal sleep-wake cycle and does not initiate voluntary actions. A person in a state of coma is described as comatose. According to the Glasgow Coma Scale though, a person with confusion is considered to be in the mildest coma.

Coma may result from a variety of conditions, including intoxication (such as illicit drug abuse, overdose or misuse of over the counter medications, prescribed medication, or controlled substances), metabolic abnormalities, central nervous system diseases, acute neurologic injuries such as strokes or herniations, hypoxia, hypothermia, hypoglycemia or traumatic injuries such as head trauma caused by falls or vehicle collisions. It may also be deliberately induced by pharmaceutical agents in order to preserve higher brain functions following brain trauma, or to save the patient from extreme pain during healing of injuries or diseases.

In order for a patient to maintain consciousness, two important neurological components must function impeccably. The first is the cerebral cortex which is the gray matter covering the outer layer of the brain, and the other is a structure located in the brainstem,

called reticular activating system (RAS or ARAS). Injury to either or both of these components is sufficient to cause a patient to experience a coma. The human cortex is a group of tight, dense, "gray matter" composed of the nucleus of the neurons whose axons then form the "white matter", and is responsible for the perception of the universe, relay of the sensory input (sensation) via the thalamic pathway, and most importantly directly or indirectly in charge of all the neurological functions, from simple reflexes to complex thinking. Reticular activating system (RAS) on the other hand is a more primitive structure in the brainstem that is tightly in connection with reticular formation (RF), a critical anatomical structure needed for maintenance of arousal and sleep-wake transitions. Reticular activating system (RAS) takes its name from the effect it has on the reticular formation, which is via its stimulation. It is therefore necessary to investigate in a comatose patient, the integrity of the bilateral cerebral cortices, as well as that of the reticular activating system (RAS).

Signs and symptoms

Generally, a patient who is unable to voluntarily open the eyes, does not have a sleep-wake cycle, is unresponsive in spite of strong tactile(painful), or verbal stimuli and who generally scores between 3 to 8[3] on the Glasgow Coma Scale is considered to be in coma.[1] Coma may have developed in humans as a response to injury to allow the body to pause bodily actions and heal the most immediate injuries before - if at all - waking. It therefore could be a compensatory state in which the body's expenditure of energy is not superfluous. The severity and mode of onset of coma depends on the underlying cause. For instance,

severe hypoglycemia (low blood sugar) or hypercapnia (increased carbon dioxide levels in the blood) initially cause mild agitation and confusion, but progress to obtundation, stupor and finally complete unconsciousness. In contrast, coma resulting from a severe traumatic brain injury or subarachnoid hemorrhage can be instantaneous. The mode of onset may therefore be indicative of the underlying cause. A state of unconsciousness lasting less than 6 hours is not by definition a coma, but a concussion, therefore a patient who loses consciousness for less than this time period should not be immediately labeled as having experienced a coma.

Diagnosis and findings

Diagnosis of coma is simple; however, diagnosing the cause of the underlying disease process often proves to be challenging. The first priority in treatment of a comatose patient is stabilization following the basic ABCs (standing for airway, breathing, and circulation).

Once a person in a coma is stable, investigations are performed to assess the underlying cause. Investigative methods are divided into physical examination findings and imaging (such as CAT scan, MRI, etc.) and special studies (EEG, etc.)

Initial assessment and evaluation

In the initial assessment of coma, it is common to gauge the level of consciousness by spontaneously exhibited actions, response to vocal stimuli ("Can you hear me?"), and painful stimuli; this is known as the AVPU (alert, vocal stimuli, painful stimuli, unresponsive) scale. More elaborate scales, such as the Glasgow Coma Scale, quantify an individual's reactions such as eye opening, movement and verbal response on a scale; Glasgow Coma Scale (GCS) is an indication of the extent of brain injury varying from 3 (indicating severe brain injury and death) to a maximum of 15 (indicating mild or no brain injury).

In those with deep unconsciousness, there is a risk of asphyxiation as the control over the muscles in the face and throat is diminished. As a result, those presenting to a hospital with coma are typically assessed for this risk ("airway management"). If the risk of asphyxiation is deemed to be high, doctors may use various devices (such as an oropharyngeal

airway, nasopharyngeal airway or endotracheal tube) to safeguard the airway.

Physical examination findings

Physical examination is critical after stabilization. It should include vital signs, a general portion dedicated to making observations about the patient's respiration (breathing pattern), body movements (if any), and of the patient's body habitus (physique); it should also include assessment of the brainstem and cortical function through special reflex tests such as the oculocephalic reflex test (doll's eyes test), oculovestibular reflex test (cold caloric test), nasal tickle, corneal reflex, and the gag reflex.

Vital signs in medicine are temperature (rectal is most accurate), blood pressure, heart rate (pulse), respiratory rate, and oxygen saturation. It should be easy to evaluate these vitals quickly in order to gain insight into a patient's metabolism, fluid status, heart function, vascular integrity, and tissue oxygenation.

Respiratory pattern (breathing rhythm) is significant and should be noted in a comatose patient. Certain stereotypical patterns of breathing have been identified including Cheyne- Stokes a form of breathing in which the patient's breathing pattern is described as alternating episodes of hyperventilation and apnea. This is a dangerous pattern and is often seen in pending herniations, extensive cortical lesions, or brainstem damage. Another pattern of breathing is apneustic breathing which is characterized by sudden pauses of inspiration and is due to a lesion of the pons. Ataxic breathing is irregular and is due to a lesion (damage) of the medulla.

Assessment of posture and body habitus is the next step. It involves general observation of the patient's positioning. There are often two stereotypical postures seen in comatose patients. Decorticate posturing is a stereotypical posturing in which the patient has arms flexed at the elbow, and arms adducted toward the body, with both legs extended. Decerebrate posturing is a stereotypical posturing in which the legs are similarly extended (stretched), but the arms are also stretched (extended at the elbow). The posturing is critical since it indicates where the damage is in the central nervous system. A decorticate posturing indicates a lesion (a point of damage) at or above the red nucleus, whereas decerebrate posturing indicates a lesion at or below the red nucleus. In other words, a decorticate lesion is closer to the cortex, as opposed to a decerebrate cortex that is closer to the brainstem.

Oculocephalic reflex also is known as the doll's eye is performed to assess the integrity of the brainstem. Patient's eyelids are gently elevated and the cornea is visualized. The patient's head is then moved to the patient's left, to observe if the eyes stay or deviate toward the patient's right; the same manoeuvre is attempted on the opposite side. If the patient's eyes move in a direction opposite to the direction of the rotation of the head, then the patient is said to have an intact brainstem. However, the failure of both eyes to move to one side can indicate damage or destruction of the affected side. In special cases, where only one eye deviates and the other does not, this often indicates a lesion (or damage) of the medial longitudinal fasciculus (MLF) which is a brainstem nerve tract. Caloric reflex test also evaluates both cortical and brainstem function; cold water is injected into one ear and the patient is observed for eye movement; if the patient's eyes slowly deviate toward the ear where the water was injected, then the brainstem is intact, however, failure to deviate toward the injected ear indicates damage of the brainstem on that side. Cortex is responsible for rapid nystagmus away from this deviated position and is often seen in patients who are conscious or merely lethargic.

An important part of the physical exam is also an assessment of the cranial nerves. Due to the unconscious status of the patient, only a limited number of the nerves can be assessed.

These include the cranial nerves number 2 (CN II), number 3 (CN III), number 5 (CN V), number 7 (CN VII), and cranial nerves 9 and 10 (CN IX, CN X). Gag reflex helps assess cranial nerves 9 and 10. Pupil reaction to light is important because it shows an intact retina, and cranial nerve number 2 (CN II); if pupils are reactive to light, then that also indicates that the cranial nerve number 3 (CN III) (or at least its parasympathetic fibres) are intact. Corneal reflex assesses the integrity of cranial nerve number 7 (CN VII), and cranial nerve number 5 (CN V). Cranial nerve number 5 (CN V), and its ophthalmic branch (V_1) are responsible for the afferent arm of the reflex, and the cranial nerve number 7 (CN VII) also known a facial nerve, is responsible for the efferent arm, causing contraction of the muscle orbicularis oculi resulting in closing of the eyes.

Pupil assessment is often a critical portion of a comatose examination, as it can give information as to the cause of the coma;

Both pupils are dilated and unreactive to light. This could be due to overdose of certain medications, hypothermia or severe anoxia (lack of oxygen).

Imaging and special tests findings

Imaging basically encompasses computed tomography (CAT or CT) scan of the brain, or MRI for example, and is performed to identify specific causes of the coma, such as hemorrhage in the brain or herniation of the brain structures. Special tests such as an EEG can also show a lot about the activity level of the cortex such as semantic processing, presence of seizures, and are important available tools not only for the assessment of the cortical activity but also for predicting the likelihood of the patient's awakening. The autonomous responses such as the Skin Conductance Response may also provide further insight on the patient's emotional processing.

History

When diagnosing any neurological condition, history and examination are fundamental. History is obtained by family, friends or EMS. The Glasgow Coma Scale is a helpful system used to examine and determine the depth of coma, track patients progress and predict outcome as best as possible. In general, a correct diagnosis can be achieved by combining findings from physical exam, imaging, and history components and will direct the appropriate therapy.

Severity and classification

Plum and Posner classify coma as either (1) supratentorial (above Tentorium cerebelli),

(2) infratentorial (below Tentorium cerebelli), or (3) metabolic or (4) diffuse. This classification is merely dependent on the position of the original damage that caused the coma, and does not correlate with severity or the prognosis. The severity of coma impairment however is categorized into several levels. Patients may or may not progress through these levels. In the first level, the brain responsiveness lessens, normal reflexes are lost, the patient no longer responds to pain and cannot hear.

The Rancho Los Amigos Scale is a complex scale that has eight separate levels, and is often used in the first few weeks or months of coma while the patient is under closer observation, and when shifts between levels are more frequent.

Prognosis

Outcomes range from recovery to death. Comas can last from several days to several weeks. In more severe cases a coma may last for over 5 weeks, while some have lasted as long as several years. After this time, some patients gradually come out of the coma, some progress to a vegetative state, and others die. Some patients who have entered a vegetative state go on to regain a degree of awareness. Others remain in a vegetative state for years or even decades (the longest recorded period being 37 years).

The outcome for coma and vegetative state depends on the cause, location, severity and extent of neurological damage. A deeper coma alone does not necessarily mean a slimmer chance of recovery, because some people in deep coma recover well while others in a so- called milder coma sometimes fail to improve.

People may emerge from a coma with a combination of physical, intellectual and psychological difficulties that need special attention. Recovery usually occurs gradually— patients acquire more and more ability to respond. Some patients never progress beyond very basic responses, but many recover full awareness. Regaining consciousness is not instant: in the first days, patients are only awake for a few minutes, and duration of time awake gradually increases. This is unlike the situation in many movies where people who awake from comas are instantly able to continue their normal lives. In reality, the coma patient awakes sometimes in a profound state of confusion, not knowing how they got there and sometimes suffering from dysarthria, the inability to articulate any speech, and with many other disabilities.

Predicted chances of recovery are variable owing to different techniques used to measure the extent of neurological damage. All the predictions are based on statistical rates with some level of chance for recovery present: a person with a low chance of recovery may still awaken. Time is the best general predictor of a chance of recovery: after 4 months of coma caused by brain damage, the chance of partial recovery is less than 15%, and the chance of full recovery is very low.

The most common cause of death for a person in a vegetative state is secondary infection such as pneumonia which can occur in patients who lie still for extended periods.

Treatment and recovery

Medical treatment

Coma is a medical emergency, and attention must first be directed to maintaining the patient's respiration and circulation, using intubation and ventilation, administration of intravenous fluids or blood and other supportive care as needed. Once a patient is stable and no longer in immediate danger, the medical staff may concentrate on maintaining the health of patient's physical state. The concentration will be directed on preventing infections such as pneumonias, bedsores (decubitus ulcers) and providing a balanced nutrition These infections may appear from the patient not being able to move around, and being confined to the bed. The nursing staff will move the patient every 2–3 hours from side to side and depending on the state of consciousness sometimes to a chair. The goal is to move the patient as much as possible to try to avoid bedsores, atelectasis and pneumonia. Pneumonia can occur from the person's inability to swallow leading to aspiration, lack of gag reflex or from the feeding tube, (aspiration pneumonia). Physical therapy may also be used to prevent contractures and orthopedic deformities that would limit recovery for those patients who emerge from coma.

A person in a coma may become restless, or seize and need special care to prevent them from hurting themselves. Medicine may be given to calm such individuals. Patients who are restless may also try to pull on tubes or dressings so soft cloth wrist restraints may be put on. Side rails on the bed should be kept up to prevent patient from falling.

Emotional challenges

Coma has a wide variety of emotional reactions from the family members of the affected patients, as well as the primary caregivers taking care of the patients. Common reactions, such as desperation, anger, frustration, and denial are possible. The focus of patient care should be on creating an amicable relationship with the family members or dependents of a comatose patient as well as creating rapport with the medical staff.

CHAPTER TWENTY-THREE

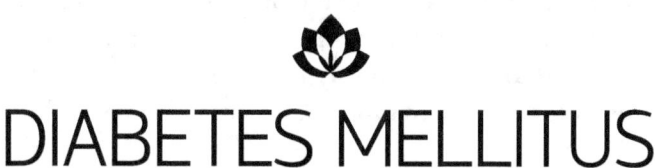

DIABETES MELLITUS

Diabetes mellitus, often simply referred to as diabetes, is a group of metabolic diseases in which a person has high blood sugar, either because the body does not produce enough insulin, or because cells do not respond to the insulin that is produced. This high blood sugar produces the classical symptoms of polyuria (frequent urination), polydipsia (increased thirst) and polyphagia (increased hunger).

There are three main types of diabetes:

Type 1 diabetes: results from the body's failure to produce insulin, and presently requires the person to inject insulin. (Also referred to as *insulin-dependent* diabetes mellitus, *IDDM* for short, and *juvenile* diabetes.)

Type 2 diabetes: results from insulin resistance, a condition in which cells fail to use insulin properly, sometimes combined with an absolute insulin deficiency. (Formerly referred to as *non-insulin-dependent* diabetes mellitus, *NIDDM* for short, and *adult-onset* diabetes.)

Gestational diabetes: is when pregnant women, who have never had diabetes before, have a high blood glucose level during pregnancy. It may precede development of type 2 DM.

Other forms of diabetes mellitus include congenital diabetes, which is due to genetic defects of insulin secretion, cystic fibrosis- related diabetes, steroid diabetes induced by high doses of glucocorticoids, and several forms of monogenic diabetes.

All forms of diabetes have been treatable since insulin became available in 1921, and type 2 diabetes may be controlled with medications. Both type 1 and 2 are chronic conditions that usually cannot be cured. Pancreas transplants have been tried with limited success in type 1 DM; gastric bypass surgery has been successful in many with morbid obesity and type 2 DM. Gestational diabetes usually resolves after Delivery. Diabetes without proper treatments can cause many complications. Acute complications include hypoglycemia, diabetic ketoacidosis, or nonketotic hyperosmolar coma. Serious long-term complications

Include cardiovascular disease, chronic renal failure, retinal damage. Adequate treatment of diabetes is thus important, as well as blood pressure control and lifestyle factors such as smoking cessation and maintaining a healthy body weight.

Classification

Most cases of diabetes mellitus fall into three broad categories: type 1, type 2, and gestational diabetes. A few other types are described. The term *diabetes*, without qualification, usually refers to diabetes *mellitus*. The rare disease diabetes insipidus has Comparison of type 1 and 2 diabetes

Type 1 diabetes

Type 1 diabetes mellitus is characterized by loss of the insulin- producing beta cells of the islets of Langerhans in the pancreas leading to insulin deficiency. This type of diabetes can be further classified as immune-mediated or idiopathic. The majority of type 1 diabetes is of the immune-mediated nature, where beta cell loss is a T-cell mediated autoimmune attack. There is no known preventive measure against type 1 diabetes, which causes approximately 10% of diabetes mellitus cases in North America and Europe. Most affected people are otherwise healthy and of a healthy weight when onset occurs. Sensitivity and responsiveness to insulin are usually normal, especially in the early stages. Type 1 diabetes can affect children or adults but was traditionally termed "juvenile diabetes" because it represents a majority of the diabetes cases in children.

Brittle diabetes, also known as unstable diabetes or labile diabetes, refers to a type of insulin-dependent diabetes characterized by dramatic and recurrent swings in glucose levels, often occurring for no apparent reason the result can be irregular and unpredictable hyperglycemias, frequently with ketosis, and sometimes serious hypoglycemia's. Brittle diabetes occurs no more frequently than in 1% to 2% of diabetics

Type 2 diabetes

Type 2 diabetes mellitus is characterized by insulin resistance which may be combined with relatively reduced insulin secretion. The defective responsiveness of body tissues to insulin is believed to involve the insulin receptor. However, the specific defects are not known. Diabetes mellitus due to a known defect are classified separately. Type 2 diabetes is the most common type.

In the early stage of type 2 diabetes, the predominant abnormality is reduced insulin sensitivity. At this stage hyperglycemia can be reversed by a variety of measures and medications that improve insulin sensitivity or reduce glucose production by the liver.

Gestational diabetes

Gestational diabetes mellitus (GDM) resembles type 2 diabetes in several respects, involving a combination of relatively inadequate insulin secretion and responsiveness. It occurs in about 2%–5% of all pregnancies and may improve or disappear after delivery.

Gestational diabetes is fully treatable but requires careful medical supervision throughout the pregnancy. About 20%–50% of affected women develop type 2 diabetes later in life.

Even though it may be transient, untreated gestational diabetes can damage the health of the fetus or mother. Risks to the baby include macrosomia (high birth weight), congenital cardiac and central nervous system anomalies, and skeletal muscle malformations. Increased fetal insulin may inhibit fetal surfactant production and cause respiratory distress syndrome. Hyperbilirubinemia may result from red blood cell destruction. In severe cases, perinatal death may occur, most commonly as a result of poor placental perfusion due to vascular impairment. Labor induction may be indicated with decreased placental function. A cesarean section may be performed if there is marked fetal distress or an increased risk of injury associated with macrosomia, such as shoulder dystocia.

Signs and symptoms

The classical symptoms of diabetes are polyuria (frequent urination), polydipsia (increased thirst) and polyphagia (increased hunger Symptoms may develop rapidly (weeks or months) in type 1 diabetes while in type 2 diabetes they usually develop much more slowly and may be subtle or absent.

Prolonged high blood glucose causes glucose absorption, which leads to changes in the shape of the lenses of the eyes, resulting in vision changes; sustained sensible glucose control usually returns the lens to its original shape. Blurred vision is a common complaint leading to a diabetes diagnosis; type 1 should always be suspected in cases of rapid vision change, whereas with type 2 change is generally more gradual, but should still be suspectedPeople (usually with type 1 diabetes) may also present with diabetic ketoacidosis, a state of metabolic dysregulation characterized by the smell of acetone; a rapid, deep breathing known asKussmaul breathing; nausea; vomiting and abdominal pain; and altered states of consciousness.

A rarer but equally severe possibility is hyperosmolar nonketotic state, which is more common in type 2 diabetes and is mainly the result of dehydration. Often, the patient has been drinking extreme amounts of sugar-containing drinks, leading to a vicious circle in regard to the water loss.

A number of skin rashes can occur in diabetes that are collectively known as diabetic dermadromes.

Causes

The cause of diabetes depends on the type.

Type 1 diabetes is partly inherited and then triggered by certain infections, with some evidence pointing at Coxsackie B4 virus.

There is a genetic element in individual susceptibility to some of these triggers which has been traced to particular HLA genotypes (i.e., the genetic "self" identifiers relied upon by the immune system). However, even in those who have inherited the susceptibility, type 1 diabetes mellitus seems to require an environmental trigger. Type 2 diabetes is due primarily to lifestyle factors and genetics

Following is a comprehensive list of other causes of diabetes:

Genetic defects of β-cell Function
Maturity onset diabetes of the young (MODY)
Mitochondrial DNA mutations
Genetic defects in insulin processing or insulin action
Defects in proinsulin conversion
Insulin gene mutations
Insulin receptor mutations
Exocrine Pancreatic Defects
Chronic pancreatitis
Pancreatectomy
Pancreatic neoplasia
Cystic fibrosis
Hemochromatosis
Fibro calculous pancreatopathy

Diagnosis

Diabetes mellitus is characterized by recurrent or persistent hyperglycemia, and is diagnosed by demonstrating any one of the following

Fasting plasma glucose level ≥ 7.0 mmol/L (126 mg/dL).

Plasma glucose ≥ 11.1 mmol/L (200 mg/dL) two hours after a 75 g oral glucose load as in a glucose tolerance test.

Symptoms of hyperglycemia and casual plasma glucose ≥ 11.1 mmol/L (200 mg/dL).

Glycated hemoglobin (Hb A1C) ≥ 6.5%.

A positive result, in the absence of unequivocal hyperglycemia, should be confirmed by a repeat of any of the above-listed methods on a different day. It is preferable to measure a fasting glucose level because of the ease of measurement and the considerable time commitment of formal glucose tolerance testing, which takes two hours to complete and offers no prognostic advantage over the fasting test. according to the current definition, two fasting glucose measurements above 126 mg/dL (7.0 mmol/L) is considered diagnostic for diabetes mellitus.

People with fasting glucose levels from 100 to 125 mg/dL (5.6 to 6.9 mmol/L) are considered to have impaired fasting glucose.

Patients with plasma glucose at or above 140 mg/dL (7.8 mmol/L), but not over 200 mg/dL (11.1 mmol/L), two hours after a 75 g oral glucose load are considered to have impaired glucose tolerance. Of these two pre-diabetic states, the latter in particular is a

major risk factor for progression to full-blown diabetes mellitus as well as cardiovascular disease.

Management

Diabetes mellitus is a chronic disease which cannot be cured except in very specific situations. Management concentrates on keeping blood sugar levels as close to normal ("euglycemia") as possible, without causing hypoglycemia. This can usually be accomplished with diet, exercise, and use of appropriate medications (insulin in the case of type 1 diabetes, oral medications as well as possibly insulin in type 2 diabetes).

Patient education, understanding, and participation is vital since the complications of diabetes are far less common and less severe in people who have well-managed blood sugar levels the goal of treatment is an HbA1C level of 6.5%, but should not be lower than that, and may be set higher. Attention is also paid to other health problems that may accelerate the deleterious effects of diabetes. These include smoking, elevated cholesterol levels, obesity, high blood pressure, and lack of regular exercise.

Lifestyle

There are roles for patient education, dietetic support, sensible exercise, with the goal of keeping both short-term and long-term blood glucose levels within acceptable bounds. In addition, given the associated higher risks of cardiovascular disease, lifestyle modifications are recommended to control blood pressure.

Medications

Oral medications

Metformin is generally recommended as a first line treatment for type 2 diabetes as there is good evidence that it decreases mortality. Routine use of aspirin however has not been found to improve outcomes in uncomplicated diabetes.

Insulin

Type 1 diabetes is typically treated with a combination of regular and NPH insulin, or synthetic insulin analogs. When insulin is used in type 2 diabetes, a long-acting formulation is usually added initially, while continuing oral medications. Doses of insulin are than increased to effect.

CHAPTER TWENTY-FOUR

ADDISON'S DISEASE & HYPOTHYROIDISM

Addison's disease (also chronic adrenal insufficiency, hypocortisolism, andhypocorticism) is a rare, chronic endocrine disorder where the adrenal glands do not produce sufficient steroid hormones (glucocorticoids and often mineralocorticoids). Lifelong, continuous treatment with steroid replacement therapy is required, with regular follow-up treatment and monitoring for other health problems

It is generally diagnosed via blood tests and medical imaging. Treatment involves replacing the absent hormones (oral hydrocortisone and fludrocortisone).

Addison's disease is named after Dr. Thomas Addison, the British physician who first described the condition in *On the Constitutional and Local Effects of Disease of the Suprarenal Capsules*(1849). The adjective "Addisonian" describes features of the condition, and patients suffering from Addison's disease While Addison's six patients in 1855 all had adrenal tuberculosis, the term "Addison's disease" does not imply an underlying disease process.

Signs and symptoms

The symptoms of Addison's disease develop insidiously, and it may take some time to be recognized. The most common symptoms are fatigue, lightheadedness upon standing or while upright, muscle weakness, fever, weight loss, difficulty in standing up, anxiety, nausea, vomiting, diarrhoea, headache, sweating, changes in mood and personality, and joint and muscle pains.

Some have marked cravings for salt or salty foods due to the urinary losses of sodium. Affected individuals may note increased tanning since adrenal insufficiency is manifested in the skin primarily by hyperpigmentation, specifically due to the decrease in cortisol and subsequent increase in ACTH levels.

Clinical signs

Low blood pressure that falls further when standing (orthostatic hypotension)

In long-standing Addison's Disease, the pinna of the ear may become calcified

Most people with primary Addison's have darkening (hyperpigmentation) of the skin, including areas not exposed to the sun; characteristic sites are skin creases (e.g. of the hands), nipple, and the inside of the cheek (buccal mucosa), also old scars may darken. This occurs because melanocyte-stimulating hormone (MSH) and adrenocorticotropic hormone (ACTH) share the same precursor molecule, Pro-opiomelanocortin (POMC). After production in anterior pituitary gland, POMC gets cleaved into Gamma-MSH, ACTH and Beta-lipotropin. The subunit ACTH undergoes further cleavage to produce Alpha-MSH, the most important MSH for skin pigmentation. In secondary and tertiary forms of Addison's, skin darkening does not occur.

Medical conditions such as type I diabetes, autoimmune thyroid disease (Hashimoto's thyroiditis and goiter)and vitiligo often occur together with Addison's (often in the setting of Autoimmune polyendocrine syndrome). Hence, symptoms and signs of any of the former conditions may also be present in the individual with Addison's.

The occurrence of Addison's Disease in someone who also has Hashimoto's thyroiditis is called Schmidt syndrome.

Addisonian crisis

An "Addisonian crisis" or "adrenal crisis" is a constellation of symptoms that indicate severe adrenal insufficiency. This may be the result of either previously undiagnosed Addison's disease, a disease process suddenly affecting adrenal function (such as adrenal hemorrhage), or an intercurrent problem (e.g. infection, trauma) in someone known to have Addison's disease. It is a medical emergency and potentially life-threatening situation requiring immediate emergency treatment.

Characteristic symptoms are:
Sudden penetrating pain in the legs, lower back or abdomen
Severe vomiting and diarrhea, resulting in dehydration
Low blood pressure
Syncope (loss of consciousness and ability to stand)
Hypoglycemia (reduced level of blood glucose)
Confusion, psychosis, slurred speech
Severe lethargy
Hyponatremia
Hyperkalemia (elevated potassium level in the blood)
Hypercalcemia (elevated calcium level in the blood)
Convulsions
Fever

Causes

Causes of adrenal insufficiency can be grouped by the way they cause the adrenals to produce insufficient cortisol. These are *adrenal dysgenesis* (the gland has not formed adequately during development), *impaired steroidogenesis* (the gland is present but is biochemically unable to produce cortisol) or *adrenal destruction* (disease processes leading to the gland being damaged).

Adrenal dysgenesis

All causes in this category are genetic, and generally very rare. These include mutations to the *SF1* transcription factor, congenital adrenal hypoplasia (AHC) due to *DAX-1* gene mutations and mutations to the ACTH receptor gene (or related genes, such as in the Triple A or Allgrove syndrome). *DAX-1* mutations may cluster in a syndrome with glycerol kinase deficiency with a number of other symptoms when*DAX-1* is deleted together with a number of other genes.

Impaired steroidogenesis

To form cortisol, the adrenal gland requires cholesterol, which is then converted biochemically into steroid hormones. Interruptions in the delivery of cholesterol include Smith-Lemli-Opitz syndrome and abetalipoproteinemia.

Of the synthesis problems, congenital adrenal hyperplasia is the most common (in various forms: 21-hydroxylase, 17α-hydroxylase, 11β-hydroxylase and 3β-hydroxysteroid dehydrogenase), lipoid CAH due to deficiency of StAR and mitochondrial DNA mutations. Some medications interfere with steroid synthesis enzymes (e.g. ketoconazole), while others accelerate the normal breakdown of hormones by the liver (e.g. rifampicin, phenytoin).

Adrenal destruction

Autoimmune adrenalitis is the most common cause of Addison's disease in the industrialized world. Autoimmune destruction of the adrenal cortex is cause by an immune reaction against the enzyme 21-hydroxylase (a phenomenon first described in 1992). This may be isolated or in the context of autoimmune polyendocrine syndrome (APS type 1 or 2), in which other hormone-producing organs such as the thyroid and pancreas may also be affected.

Adrenal destruction is also a feature of adrenoleukodystrophy (ALD), and when the adrenal glands are involved in metastasis (seeding of cancer cells from elsewhere in the body, especially lung), hemorrhage (e.g. in Waterhouse-Frederiksen syndrome or antiphospholipid syndrome), particular infections (tuberculosis histoplasmosis, coccidioidomycosis), deposition of abnormal protein in amyloidosis.

Diagnosis

Routine investigations may show: Hypercalcemia

Hypoglycemia, low blood sugar (worse in children due to loss of glucocorticoid's glucogenic effects)

Hyponatremia (low blood sodium levels), due to the kidney's inability to excrete free water in the absence of sufficient cortisol, and also the effect of Corticotropin-releasing hormone to stimulate secretion of ADH. That hyponatremia occurs even when the adrenal insufficiency is due to pituitary disease (in which aldosterone deficiency is *not* a feature), underscores the fact that hyponatremia in Addison's disease is not due to lack of aldosterone.

Hyperkalemia (raised blood potassium levels), due to loss of production of the hormone aldosterone Eosinophilia and lymphocytosis (increased number of eosinophils or lymphocytes, two types of white blood cells) Metabolic acidosis (increased blood acidity), also due to loss of the hormone aldosterone because sodium reabsorption in the distal tubule is linked with acid/hydrogen ion (H+) secretion. Low levels of aldosterone stimulation of the renal distal tubule lead to sodium wasting in the urine and H+ retention in the serum.

In suspected cases of Addison's disease, one needs to demonstrate that adrenal hormone levels are low even after appropriate stimulation (called the ACTH stimulation test) with synthetic pituitary ACTH hormone tetracosactide. Two tests are performed, the

short and the long test.

The short test compares blood cortisol levels before and after 250 micrograms of tetracosactide (IM/IV) is given. If, one hour later, plasma cortisol exceeds 170 nmol/L and has risen by at least 330 nmol/L to at least 690 nmol/L, adrenal failure is excluded. If the short test is abnormal, the long test is used to differentiate between primary adrenal insufficiency and secondary adrenocortical insufficiency.

The long test uses 1 mg tetracosactide (IM). Blood is taken 1, 4, 8, and 24 hours later. Normal plasma cortisol level should reach 1000 nmol/L by 4 hours. In primary Addison's disease, the cortisol level is reduced at all stages whereas in secondary corticoadrenal insufficiency, a delayed but normal response is seen.

Other tests that may be performed to distinguish between various causes of hypoadrenalism are renin and adrenocorticotropic hormone levels, as well as medical imaging - usually in the form of ultrasound, computed tomography or magnetic resonance imaging (MRI).

Maintenance

Treatment for Addison's disease involves replacing the missing cortisol, sometimes in the form of hydrocortisone tablets, or prednisone tablets in a dosing regimen that mimics the physiological concentrations of cortisol. Alternatively, one quarter as much prednisolone may be used for equal glucocorticoid effect as hydrocortisone. Treatment must usually be continued for life. In addition, many patients require fludrocortisone as replacement for the missing aldosterone. Caution must be exercised when the person with Addison's disease becomes unwell with infection, has surgery or other trauma, or becomes pregnant. In such instances, their replacement glucocorticoids, whether in the form of hydrocortisone, prednisone, prednisolone, or other equivalent, often need to be increased. Inability to take oral medication may prompt hospital attendance to receive steroids intravenously. People with Addison's are often advised to carry information on them (e.g. in the form of a Medic Alert bracelet) for the attention of emergency medical services personnel who might need to attend to their needs.

Epidemiology

The frequency rate of Addison's disease in the human population is sometimes estimated at roughly 1 in 100,000. Some research and information sites put the number closer to 40-60 cases per 1 million population. (1/25,000-1/16,600) (Determining accurate numbers for Addison's is problematic at best and some incidence figures are thought to be underestimates. Addison's can afflict persons of any age, gender, or ethnicity, but it typically presents in adults between 30 and 50 years of age. Research has shown no significant predispositions based on ethnicity.

Prognosis

With proper medication, patients can expect to live a healthy and normal life. A person with adrenal insufficiency should always carry identification stating their condition in case of an emergency. The card should alert emergency personnel about the need to inject 100 mg of cortisol if its bearer is found severely injured or unable to answer questions. The card should also include the doctor's name and telephone number and the name and telephone number of the nearest relative to be notified. When traveling, a needle, syringe, and an injectable form of cortisol should be carried for emergencies. A person with Addison's disease also should know how to increase medication during periods of stress or mild upper respiratory infections. Immediate medical attention is needed when severe infections, vomiting, or diarrhea occur, as these conditions can precipitate an Addisonian crisis. A patient who is vomiting may require injections of hydrocortisone, since oral hydrocortisone supplements cannot be adequately metabolized.

HYPOTHYROIDISM

Hypothalamus

Results when the hypothalamus fails to produce sufficient thyrotropin-releasing hormone (TRH). TRH prompts the pituitary gland to produce thyroid-stimulating hormone (TSH). Hence may also be termed *hypothalamic-pituitary-axis hypothyroidism*. It accounts for less than 5% of hypothyroidism cases.

Signs and symptoms

Early hypothyroidism is often asymptomatic and can have very mild symptoms. *Subclinical hypothyroidism* is a state of normal thyroid hormone levels, thyroxine (T4) and triiodothyronine (T3), with mild elevation of thyrotropin, thyroid-stimulating hormone (TSH). With higher TSH levels and low free T4 levels, symptoms become more readily apparent in *clinical* (or overt) *hypothyroidism*.

Hypothyroidism can be associated with the following symptoms:
Poor muscle tone (muscle hypotonia)
Fatigue
Any form of menstrual irregularity and fertility problems
Hyperprolactinemia and galactorrhea
Elevated serum cholesterol
Cold intolerance, increased sensitivity to cold
Constipation

Rapid thoughts
Depression
Muscle cramps and joint pain
Thin, brittle fingernails
Coarse hair
Paleness
Decreased sweating
Dry, itchy skin
Weight gain and water retention
Bradycardia (low heart rate – fewer than sixty beats per minute)
Goiter

Slow speech and a hoarse, breaking voice – deepening of the voice can also be noticed, caused by Reinke's Edema.

Dry puffy skin, especially on the face
Thinning of the outer third of the eyebrows (sign of Hertoghe)
Abnormal menstrual cycles
Low basal body temperature
Thyroid-Related Depression

Anemia caused by impaired hemoglobin synthesis (decreased EPO levels), impaired intestinal iron and folate absorption or B_{12} deficiency from pernicious anemia

Difficulty swallowing
Shortness of breath with a shallow and slow respiratory pattern
Increased need for sleep
Irritability and mood instability

Yellowing of the skin due to impaired conversion of beta-carotene to vitamin A (keratoderma)

Impaired renal function with decreased glomerular filtration rate
Acute psychosis (myxedema madness) (a rare presentation of hypothyroidism)
Decreased libido in men due to impairment of testicular testosterone synthesis
Decreased sense of taste and smell (anosmia)
Puffy face, hands and feet (late, less common symptoms)
Gynecomastia
Deafness
Subclinical hypothyroidism

Subclinical hypothyroidism occurs when thyrotropin (TSH) levels are elevated but thyroxine (T_4) and triiodothyronine (T_3) levels are normal. In primary hypothyroidism, TSH levels are high and T_4 and T_3 levels are low. TSH usually increases when T_4 and T_3 levels drop. TSH prompts the thyroid gland to make more hormone. In subclinical hypothyroidism, TSH is elevated but below the limit representing overt hypothyroidism. The levels of the active hormones will be within the laboratory reference ranges.

Epidemiology

About three percent of the general population has hypothyroidism. Estimates of subclinical hypothyroidism range between 3–8%, increasing with age; incidence is more common in women than in men.

Causes

Iodine deficiency is the most common cause of hypothyroidism worldwide. In iodine-replete individuals' hypothyroidism is frequently caused by Hashimoto's thyroiditis, or otherwise as a result of either an absent thyroid gland or a deficiency in stimulating hormones from the hypothalamus or pituitary.

Factors such as iodine deficiency or exposure to iodine-131 from nuclear fallout, which is absorbed by the thyroid gland like regular iodide and destroys its cells, can increase the risk.

Congenital hypothyroidism is very rare accounting for approximately 0.2‰ and can have several causes such as thyroid aplasia or defects in the hormone metabolism. Thyroid hormone insensitivity (most often T3 receptor defect) also falls into this category although in this condition the levels of thyroid hormones may be normal or even markedly elevated.

Hypothyroidism can result from postpartum thyroiditis, a condition that affects about 5% of all women within a year of giving birth

The first phase is typically hyperthyroidism; the thyroid then either returns to normal, or a woman develops hypothyroidism. Of those women who experience hypothyroidism associated with postpartum thyroiditis, one in five will develop permanent hypothyroidism requiring life-long treatment.

Hypothyroidism can result from de Quervain's thyroiditis, which, in turn, is often caused by having a bad flu that enters and destroys part, or all, the thyroid.

Hypothyroidism can also result from sporadic inheritance, sometimes autosomal recessive

Hypothyroidism is also a relatively common disease in domestic dogs, with some specific breeds having a definite predisposition.

Temporary hypothyroidism can be due to the Wolff-Chaikoff effect. A very high intake of iodine can be used to temporarily treat hyperthyroidism, especially in an emergency situation. Although iodide is a substrate for thyroid hormones, high levels reduce iodide organification in the thyroid gland, decreasing hormone production.

The antiarrhythmic agent amiodarone can cause hyper- or hypothyroidism due to its high iodine content.

Hypothyroidism can be caused by lithium-based mood stabilizers, usually used to treat bipolar disorder (previously known as manic depression). In fact, lithium has occasionally been used to treat hyperthyroidism. Other drugs that may produce hypothyroidism include interferon alpha, interleukin-2, and thalidomide.

Diagnosis

The only validated test to diagnose primary hypothyroidism, is to measure thyroid- stimulating hormone (TSH) and free thyroxine (T4). However, these levels can be affected by non-thyroidal illnesses.

High levels of TSH indicate that the thyroid is not producing sufficient levels of thyroid hormone (mainly as thyroxine (T_4) and smaller amounts of triiodothyronine (T_3)). However, measuring just TSH fails to diagnose secondary and tertiary hypothyroidism, thus leading to the following suggested blood testing if the TSH is normal and hypothyroidism is still suspected:

Free triiodothyronine (fT_3)
Free levothyroxine (fT_4)
Total T_3
Total T_4
Additionally, the following measurements may be needed:
Free T_3 from 24-hour urine catch
  Antithyroid antibodies — for evidence of autoimmune diseases that may be damaging the thyroid gland
Serum cholesterol — which may be elevated in hypothyroidism
Prolactin — as a widely available test of pituitary function
Testing for anemia, including ferritin
Basal body temperature

Misdiagnosis is common in hypothyroidism, with many patterns of dysfunction failing to be identified by most laboratory tests: normal TSH, T3 and T4 levels are expected in many types of thyroid dysfunction especially those associated with increased stress

Treatment

Hypothyroidism is treated with the levorotatory forms of thyroxine (levothyroxine) (L-T_4) and triiodothyronine (liothyronine) (L-T_3). Synthroid is the most common name form of the pill Levothyroxine. Synthroid is also the most common pill prescribed by doctors that has the synthetic thyroid hormone in it. This medicine can improve symptoms of thyroid deficiency such as slow speech, lack of energy, weight gain, hair loss, dry skin, and feeling cold. It also helps to treat goiter. It is also used to treat some kinds of thyroid cancer along with surgery and other medicines. Both synthetic and animal-derived thyroid tablets are available and can be prescribed for patients in need of additional thyroid hormone. Thyroid hormone is taken daily, and doctors can monitor blood levels to help assure proper dosing.

Levothyroxine is best taken 30–60 minutes before breakfast, as some food can diminish absorption. Compared to water, coffee reduces absorption of levothyroxine by about 30 percent. Some patients might appear to be resistant to levothyroxine, when in fact they do not properly absorb the tablets - a problem which is solved by pulverizing the medication. There are several different treatment protocols in thyroid-replacement therapy:

T_4 only

This treatment involves supplementation of levothyroxine alone, in a synthetic form. It is currently the standard treatment in mainstream medicine.

T_4 and T_3 in combination

This treatment protocol involves administering both synthetic L-T_4 and L-T_3 simultaneously in combination.

Desiccated thyroid extract

Desiccated thyroid extract is an animal-based thyroid extract, most commonly from a porcine source. It is also a combination therapy, containing natural forms of L-T_4 and L-T_3.

Subclinical hypothyroidism

There is a range of opinion on the biochemical and symptomatic point at which to treat with levothyroxine, the typical treatment for overt hypothyroidism.

Reference ranges have been debated as well. As of 2003, the American Association of Clinical Endocrinologists (ACEE) considers 0.3–3.0 mIU/L within normal range.

There is always the risk of overtreatment and hyperthyroidism.

Alternative treatments

Compounded slow-release T3 has been suggested for use in combination with T4, which proponents argue will mitigate many of the symptoms of functional hypothyroidism and improve quality of life. This is still controversial and is rejected by the conventional medical establishment.

Hypothyroidism and Diet

This condition affects the immune system and metabolism. There are a number of supplementary vitamins and minerals specifically designed to support deficiencies in both and sufferers can mistakenly take them believing them to be beneficial. However, it is important that these should never be self-prescribed since they can directly impact the effectiveness of thyroxine (usually through preventing its absorption).

These are:
Calcium
Soya
Iron (includes Iron rich foods such as Broccoli)
Iodine (includes Kelp tablets)

Selenium (includes natural sources such as sea food)
Magnesium
Zinc
Caffeine

CHAPTER TWENTY-FIVE

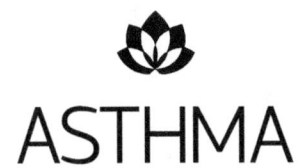

ASTHMA

Asthma (from the Greek ἄσθμα, ásthma, "panting") is the
common chronic inflammatory disease of the airways characterized by variable and recurring symptoms, reversible airflow obstruction, and bronchospasm. Symptoms
include wheezing, coughing, chest tightness, and shortness of breath Asthma is clinically classified according to the frequency of symptoms, forced expiratory volume in 1 second (FEV1), and peak expiratory flow rate. Asthma may also be classified as atopic (extrinsic) or non-atopic (intrinsic).

It is thought to be caused by a combination of genetic and environmental factors. Treatment of acute symptoms is usually with an inhaled short-acting beta-2 agonist (such as salbutamol). Symptoms can be prevented by avoiding triggers, such as allergens
and irritants, and by inhaling corticosteroids. Leukotriene antagonists are less effective than corticosteroids and thus less preferred.

Its diagnosis is usually made based on the pattern of symptoms and/or response to therapy over time. The prevalence of asthma has increased significantly since the 1970s. As of 2010, 300 million people were affected worldwide. In 2009 asthma caused 250,000 deaths globally. Despite this, with proper control of asthma with step down therapy, prognosis is generally good.

Classification
Clinical classification of severity
Severity in patients
≥ 12 years of age
Symptom frequency
Nighttime symptoms
%$FEV_1$of
predicted
FEV_1Variability
Use of short-acting beta$_2$agonist for symptom control (not for prevention of EIB)
Intermittent
≤2 per week
≤2 per month
≥80%
<20%
≤2 days per week
Mild persistent
>2 per week but not daily
3-4 per month
≥80%
20–30%
>2 days/week but not daily

Moderate persistent
Daily
>1 per week but not nightly
60–80%
>30%
Daily
Severe persistent
Throughout the day
Frequent (often 7x/week)
<60%
>30%
Several times per day

Asthma is clinically classified according to the frequency of symptoms, forced expiratory volume in 1 second (FEV_1), and peak expiratory flow rate. Asthma may also be classified as atopic (extrinsic) or non-atopic (intrinsic), based on whether symptoms are precipitated by allergens (atopic) or not (non-atopic).

While asthma is classified based on severity, at the moment there is no clear method for classifying different subgroups of asthma beyond this system. Within the classifications described above, although the cases of asthma respond to the same treatment differs, thus it is clear that the cases within a classification have significant differences. Finding ways to identify subgroups that respond well to different types of treatments is a current critical goal of asthma research.

Although asthma is a chronic obstructive condition, it is not considered as a part of chronic obstructive pulmonary disease as this term refers specifically to combinations of disease that are irreversible such as bronchiectasis, chronic bronchitis, and emphysema. Unlike these diseases, the airway obstruction in asthma is usually reversible; however, if left untreated, the chronic inflammation of the lungs during asthma can become irreversible obstruction due to airway remodeling. In contrast to emphysema, asthma affects the bronchi, not the alveoli.

Brittle asthma

Brittle asthma is a term used to describe two types of asthma, distinguishable by recurrent, severe attacks. Type 1 brittle asthma refers to disease with wide peak flow variability, despite intense medication. Type 2 brittle asthma describes background well-controlled asthma, with sudden severe exacerbations.

Asthma attack

An acute asthma exacerbation is commonly referred to as an *asthma attack*. The classic symptoms are shortness of breath, wheezing, and chest tightness.[19]While these are the primary symptoms of asthma, some people present primarily with coughing, and in severe cases, air motion may be significantly impaired such that no wheezing is heard.

Signs which occur during an asthma attack include the use of accessory muscles of respiration (sternocleidomastoid and scalene muscles of the neck), there may be

a paradoxical pulse (a pulse that is weaker during inhalation and stronger during

exhalation), and over-inflation of the chest. A blue color of the skin and nails may occur from lack of oxygen.

In a mild exacerbation the peak expiratory flow rate (PEFR) is ≥200 L/min or ≥50% of the predicted best. Moderate is defined as between 80 and 200 L/min or 25% and 50% of the predicted best while severe is defined as ≤ 80 L/min or ≤25% of the predicted best.

Insufficient levels of vitamin D are linked with severe asthma attacks.

Status asthmaticus

Status asthmaticus is an acute exacerbation of asthma that does not respond to standard treatments of bronchodilators and steroids. Nonselective beta blockers (such as Timolol) have caused fatal status asthmaticus.

Exercise induced

A diagnosis of asthma is common among top athletes. One survey of participants in the 1996 Summer Olympic Games, in Atlanta, Georgia, U.S., showed that 15% had been diagnosed with asthma, and that 10% were on asthma medication.

There appears to be a relatively high incidence of asthma in sports such as cycling, mountain biking, and long-distance running, and a relatively lower incidence in weightlifting and diving. It is unclear how much of these disparities are from the effects of training in the sport. Exercise induced asthma can be treated with the use of a short-acting beta2 agonist.

Occupational

Asthma as a result of (or worsened by) workplace exposures is a commonly reported occupational respiratory disease. Still most cases of occupational asthma are not reported or are not recognized as such. Estimates by the American Thoracic Society (2004) suggest that 15–23% of new-onset asthma cases in adults are work related. In one study monitoring workplace asthma by occupation, the highest percentage of cases occurred

among operators, fabricators, and laborers (32.9%), followed by managerial and professional specialists (20.2%), and in technical, sales, and administrative support jobs (19.2%). Most cases were associated with the manufacturing (41.4%) and services (34.2%) industries Animal proteins, enzymes, flour, natural rubber latex, and certain reactive chemicals are commonly associated with work-related asthma. When recognized, these hazards can be mitigated, dropping the risk of disease.

Signs and symptoms

Common symptoms of asthma include wheezing, shortness of breath, chest tightness

and coughing. Symptoms are often worse at night or in the early morning, or in response to exercise or cold air. Some people with asthma only rarely experience symptoms, usually in response to triggers, here as other may have marked persistent airflow obstruction.

Gastro-esophageal reflux disease

Gastro-esophageal reflux disease coexists with asthma in 80% of people with asthma, with similar symptoms. This is due to increased lung pressures, promoting bronchoconstriction, and through chronic aspiration.

Sleep disorders

Due to altered anatomy of the respiratory tract: increased upper airway adipose deposition, altered pharynx skeletal morphology, and extension of the pharyngeal airway; leading to upper airway collapse.

Causes

Asthma is caused by environmental and genetic factors. These factors influence how severe asthma is and how well it responds to medication. The interaction is complex and not fully understood. Studying the prevalence of asthma and related diseases such

as eczema and hay fever have yielded important clues about some key risk factors. The strongest risk factor for developing asthma is a history of atopic disease; this increases one's risk of hay fever by up to 5x and the risk of asthma by 3-4x. In children between the ages of 3-14, a positive skin test for allergies and an increase in immunoglobulin E increases the chance of having asthma. In adults, the more allergens one reacts positively to in a skin test, the higher the odds of having asthma.

Because much allergic asthma is associated with sensitivity to indoor allergens and because Western styles of housing favor greater exposure to indoor allergens, much attention has focused on increased exposure to these allergens in infancy and early childhood as a primary cause of the rise in asthma. Primary prevention studies aimed at the aggressive reduction of airborne allergens in a home with infants have shown mixed findings. Strict reduction of dust mite allergens, for example, reduces the risk of allergic sensitization to dust mites, and modestly reduces the risk of developing asthma up until the age of 8 years old.

However, studies also showed that the effects of exposure to cat and dog allergens worked in the converse fashion; exposure during the first year of life was found to *reduce* the risk of allergic sensitization and of developing asthma later in life.

The inconsistency of this data has inspired research into other facets of Western society and their impact upon the prevalence of asthma. One subject that appears to show a strong correlation is the development of asthma and obesity. In the United Kingdom and United States, the rise in asthma prevalence has echoed an almost epidemic rise in the prevalence of obesity. In Taiwan, symptoms of allergies and airway hyper-reactivity increased in correlation with each 20% increase in body-mass index. Several factors associated with obesity may play a role in the pathogenesis of asthma, including decreased respiratory function due to a buildup of adipose tissue (fat) and the fact that adipose tissue leads to a pro-inflammatory state, which has been associated with non-eosinophilic asthma. Asthma has been associated with Churg–Strauss syndrome, and individuals with immunologically mediated urticaria may also experience systemic symptoms with generalized urticaria,

rhino-conjunctivitis, or laryngeal and gastrointestinal symptoms, asthma, and, at worst, anaphylaxis. Additionally, adult-onset asthma has been associated with

periocular xanthogranulomas.

Environmental

Many environmental risk factors have been associated with asthma development and morbidity in children. Recent studies show a relationship between exposure to air pollutants (e.g. from traffic) and childhood asthma. This research finds that both the occurrence of the disease and exacerbation of childhood asthma are affected by outdoor air pollutants. High levels of endotoxin exposure may contribute to asthma risk Viral respiratory infections are not only one of the leading triggers of an exacerbation but may increase one's risk of developing asthma especially in young children.

Respiratory infections such as rhinovirus, *Chlamydia pneumoniae* and *Bordetella pertussis* are correlated with asthma exacerbations.

Psychological stress has long been suspected of being an asthma trigger, but only in recent decades has convincing scientific evidence substantiated this hypothesis. Rather than stress directly causing the asthma symptoms, it is thought that stress modulates the immune system to increase the magnitude of the airway inflammatory response to allergens and irritants. Beta blocker medications such as metoprolol may trigger asthma in those who are susceptible.

Tobacco

Maternal tobacco smoking during pregnancy and after delivery is associated with a greater risk of asthma-like symptoms, wheezing, and respiratory infections during childhood.

Low air quality, from traffic pollution or high ozone levels, has been repeatedly associated with increased asthma morbidity and has a suggested association with asthma development that needs further research.

Hygiene hypothesis

Antibiotic use early in life has been linked to development of asthma in several examples; it is thought that antibiotics make children who are predisposed to atopic immune responses susceptible to development of asthma because they modify gut flora, and thus the immune system (as described by the hygiene hypothesis). The hygiene hypothesis (see below) is

a hypothesis about the cause of asthma and other allergic disease, and is supported by epidemiologic data for asthma. All of these things may negatively affect exposure to beneficial bacteria and other immune system modulators that are important during development, and thus may cause an increased risk for asthma and allergy.

Caesarean sections have been associated with asthma, possibly because of modifications to the immune system (as described by the hygiene hypothesis).

Volatile organic compounds

Observational studies have found that indoor exposure to volatile organic

compounds (VOCs) may be one of the triggers of asthma, however experimental studies have not confirmed these observations. Even VOC exposure at low levels has been associated with an increase in the risk of pediatric asthma. Because there are so many VOCs in the air, measuring total VOC concentrations in the indoor environment may not represent the exposure of individual compounds. Exposure to VOCs is associated with an increase in the IL-4 producing Th2 cells and a reduction in IFN-γ producing Th1 cells. Thus, the mechanism of action of VOC exposure may be allergic sensitization mediated by a Th2 cell phenotype. Different individual variations in discomfort, from no response to excessive response, were seen in one of the studies. These variations may be due to the development of tolerance during exposure. Another study has concluded that formaldehyde may cause asthma-like symptoms. Low VOC emitting materials should be used while doing repairs or renovations which decreases the symptoms related to asthma caused by VOCs and formaldehyde. In another study "the indoor concentration of aliphatic compounds (C8-C11), butanol's, and 2,2,4-trimethyl 1,3-pentanediol tributyrate (TXIB) was significantly elevated in newly painted dwellings. The total indoor VOC was about 100 micrograms/m3 higher in

dwellings painted in the last year". The author concluded that some VOCs may cause inflammatory reactions in the airways and may be the reason for asthmatic symptoms.

Phthalates

There is a significant association between asthma-like symptoms (wheezing) among preschool children and the concentration of DEHP (phthalates) in indoor environment. DEHP (di-methylphenyl phthalate) is a plasticizer that is commonly used in building material. The hydrolysis product of DEHP (di-ethylhexyl phthalate) is MEHP (Mono-ethylhexyl phthalate) which mimics the prostaglandins and thromboxane's in the airway leading to symptoms related to asthma. Another mechanism that has been studied regarding phthalates causation of asthma is that high phthalates level can "modulate the murine immune response to a coallergen". Asthma can develop in the adults who come in contact with heated PVC fumes. Two main type of phthalates, namely n-butyl benzyl phthalate (BBzP) and di(2-ethylhexyl) phthalate (DEHP), have been associated between the concentration of polyvinyl chloride (PVC) used as flooring and the dust concentrations. Water leakage were associated more with BBzP, and buildings construction were associated with high concentrations of DEHP. Asthma has been shown to have a relationship with plaster wall materials and wall-to wall carpeting. The onset of asthma was also related to the floor– leveling plaster at home. Therefore, it is important to understand the health aspect of these materials in the indoor surfaces.

Genetic

Over 100 genes have been associated with asthma in at least one genetic

association study. However, such studies must be repeated to ensure the findings are not due to chance. Through the end of 2005, 25 genes had been associated with asthma in six or more separate populations:

GSTM1
IL10
CTLA-4
SPINK5
LTC4S
LTA
GRPA
NOD1
CC16
GSTP1
STAT6
NOS1
CCL5
TBXA2R
TGFB1
IL4
IL13
CD14
ADRB2 (β-2 adrenergic receptor)
HLA-DRB1

HLA-DQB1
TNF
FCER1B
IL4R
ADAM33

Many of these genes are related to the immune system or to modulating inflammation. However, even among this list of highly replicated genes associated with asthma, the results have not been consistent among all of the populations that have been tested. This indicates that these genes are not associated with asthma under every condition, and that

researchers need to do further investigation to figure out the complex interactions that cause asthma. One theory is that asthma is a collection of several diseases, and that genes might have a role in only subsets of asthma for example, one group of genetic differences (single nucleotide polymorphisms in 17q21) was associated with asthma that develops in childhood.

Gene–environment interactions
CD14-endotoxin interaction based on CD14 SNP C-159T
Endotoxin levels
CC genotype
TT genotype
High exposure
Low risk
High risk
Low exposure
High risk
Low risk

Research suggests that some genetic variants may only cause asthma when they are combined with specific environmental exposures, and otherwise may not be risk factors for asthma.

The genetic trait, CD14 single nucleotide polymorphism (SNP) C-159T and exposure to endotoxin (a bacterial product) are a well-replicated example of a gene-environment

interaction that is associated with asthma. Endotoxin exposure varies from person to person and can come from several environmental sources, including environmental tobacco smoke, dogs, and farms. Researchers have found that risk for asthma changes based on a person's genotype at CD14 C-159T and level of endotoxin exposure.

Exacerbation

Some individuals will have stable asthma for weeks or months and then suddenly develop an episode of acute asthma. Different asthmatic individuals react differently to various factors. However, most individuals can develop severe exacerbation of asthma from several triggering agents. Home factors that can lead to exacerbation include dust, house mites, animal dander (especially cat and dog hair), cockroach allergens and molds at any given home Perfumes are a common cause of acute attacks in females and children.

Both virus and bacterial infections of the upper respiratory tract infection can worsen asthma.

Hygiene hypothesis

One theory for the cause of the increase in asthma prevalence worldwide is the "hygiene hypothesis"—that the rise in the prevalence of allergies and asthma is a direct and unintended result of reduced exposure to a wide variety of different bacteria and virus types in modern societies, or modern hygienic practices preventing childhood infections. Children living in less hygienic environments (East Germany vs. West Germany, families with many children, day care environments) tend to have lower incidences of asthma and allergic diseases. This seems to run counter to the logic that viruses are often causative agents in exacerbation of asthma. Additionally, other studies have shown that viral infections of the lower airway may in some cases *induce* asthma, as a history of bronchiolitis or croup in early childhood is a predictor of asthma risk in later life. Studies which show that upper respiratory tract infections are protective against asthma risk also tend to show that lower respiratory tract infections conversely tend to increase the risk of asthma.

Socioeconomic factors

The incidence of asthma is highest among low-income populations worldwide. Asthma deaths are most common in low- and middle-income countries, and in the Western world, it is found in those low-income neighborhoods whose populations consist of large percentages of ethnic minorities. Additionally, asthma has been strongly associated with the presence of cockroaches in living quarters; these insects are more likely to be found in those same neighborhoods.

Most likely due to income and geography, the incidence of and treatment quality for asthma varies among different racial groups. The prevalence of "severe persistent" asthma is also greater in low-income communities than those with better access to treatment.

Diagnosis
   Severity of acute asthma exacerbations
   Near-fatal asthma
   High $PaCO_2$ and/or requiring mechanical ventilation
   Life threatening asthma
   Any one of the following in a person with severe asthma: -
   Clinical signs
   Measurements
   Altered level of consciousness
   Peak flow < 33%
   Exhaustion   Oxygen saturation < 92%
   Arrhythmia PaO_2 < 8 kPa
   Low blood pressure   "Normal" $PaCO_2$
   Cyanosis
   Silent chest
   Poor respiratory effort
   Any one of: -
   Peak flow 33-50%
   Acute severe asthma   Respiratory rate ≥ 25 breaths per minute
   Heart rate ≥ 110 beats per minute
   Unable to complete sentences in one breath
   Worsening symptoms
   Moderate asthma exacerbation Peak flow 80%-50% best or predicted
   No features of acute severe asthma

Obstruction of the lumen of the bronchiole by mucoid exudate, goblet cell metaplasia, epithelial basement membrane thickening and severe inflammation of bronchiole in a patient with asthma.

There is currently not a precise physiologic, immunologic, or histologic test for diagnosing asthma. The diagnosis is usually made based on the pattern of symptoms (airways obstruction and hyperresponsiveness) and/or response to therapy (partial or complete reversibility) over time. The British Thoracic Society determines a diagnosis of asthma using a 'response to therapy' approach. If the patient responds to treatment, then this is considered to be a confirmation of the diagnosis of asthma. The response measured is the reversibility of airway obstruction after treatment. Airflow in the airways is measured with

a peak flow meter or spirometer, and the following diagnostic criteria are used by the British Thoracic Society:

≥20% difference on at least three days in a week for at least two weeks;

≥20% improvement of peak flow following treatment, for example:

10 minutes of inhaled β-agonist (e.g., salbutamol);

six weeks of inhaled corticosteroid (e.g., beclomethasone);

14 days of 30 mg prednisolone.

≥20% decrease in peak flow following exposure to a trigger (e.g., exercise).

In contrast, the US National Asthma Education and Prevention Program (NAEPP) uses a 'symptom patterns' approach. Their guidelines for the diagnosis and management of asthma state that a diagnosis of asthma begins by assessing if any of the following list of indicators is present. While the indicators are not sufficient to support a diagnosis of asthma, the presence of multiple key indicators increases the probability of a diagnosis of asthma. Spirometry is needed to establish a diagnosis of asthma.

Wheezing—high-pitched whistling sounds when breathing out—especially in children. (Lack of wheezing and a normal chest examination do not exclude asthma.)

history of any of the following:

Cough, worse particularly at night

Recurrent wheeze

Recurrent difficulty in breathing

Recurrent chest tightness

Symptoms occur or worsen in the presence of:

Exercise

Viral infection

Animals with fur or hair

House-dust mites (in mattresses, pillows, upholstered furniture, carpets)

Mold

Smoke (tobacco, wood)

Pollen

Changes in weather

Strong emotional expression (laughing or crying hard)

Airborne chemicals or dusts

Menstrual cycles

Symptoms occur or worsen at night, awakening the patient

The latest guidelines from the U.S. National Asthma Education and Prevention Program (NAEPP) recommend spirometry at the time of initial diagnosis, after treatment is initiated and symptoms are stabilized, whenever control of symptoms deteriorates, and every 1 or 2 years on a regular basis. The NAEPP guidelines do not recommend testing peak expiratory flow as a regular screening method because it is more variable than spirometry. However, testing peak flow at rest (or baseline) and after exercise can be helpful, especially in young patients who may experience only exercise-induced asthma. It may also be useful for daily self-monitoring and for checking the effects of new medications. Peak flow readings can be charted together with a record of symptoms or use peak flow-charting software. This allows patients to track their peak flow readings and pass information back to their doctor or nurse.

Differential diagnosis

Differential diagnoses include: Infants and Children

Upper airway diseases

Allergic rhinitis and allergic sinusitis

Obstructions involving large airways

Foreign body in trachea or bronchus

Vocal cord dysfunction

Vascular rings or laryngeal webs

Laryngotracheomalacia, tracheal stenosis, or Broncho stenosis

Enlarged lymph nodes or tumor

Obstructions involving small airways
Viral bronchiolitis or obliterative bronchiolitis
Cystic fibrosis
Bronchopulmonary dysplasia
Heart disease
Other causes
Recurrent cough not due to asthma
> Aspiration from swallowing mechanism dysfunction or gastroesophageal reflux

Medication induced
Adults
COPD (e.g., chronic bronchitis or emphysema)
Congestive heart failure
Pulmonary embolism
Mechanical obstruction of the airways (benign and malignant tumors)
Pulmonary infiltration with eosinophilia
> Cough secondary to drugs (e.g., angiotensin-converting enzyme (ACE) inhibitors)

Vocal cord dysfunction

Before diagnosing asthma, alternative possibilities should be considered such as the use of known bronchoconstrictors (substances that cause narrowing of the airways, e.g.

certain anti-inflammatory agents or beta-blockers). Among elderly people, the presenting symptom may be fatigue, cough, or difficulty breathing, all of which may be erroneously attributed to Chronic obstructive pulmonary disease (COPD), congestive heart failure, or simple aging.

Chronic obstructive pulmonary disease

Chronic obstructive pulmonary disease can coexist with asthma and can occur as a complication of chronic asthma. After the age of 65 most people with obstructive airway disease will have asthma and COPD. In this setting, COPD can be differentiated by increased airway neutrophils, abnormally increased wall thickness, and increased smooth muscle in the bronchi. However, this level of investigation is not performed due to COPD and asthma sharing similar principles of management: corticosteroids, long acting beta agonists, and smoking cessation. It closely resembles asthma in symptoms, is correlated with more exposure to cigarette smoke, an older age, less symptom reversibility after bronchodilator administration (as measured by spirometry), and decreased likelihood of family history of atopy

Others

The term "atopy" was coined to describe this triad of atopic eczema, allergic rhinitis and asthma. Pulmonary aspiration, whether direct due to dysphagia (swallowing disorder) or indirect (due to acid reflux), can show similar symptoms to asthma. However, with aspiration, fevers might also indicate aspiration pneumonia. Direct aspiration (dysphagia) can be diagnosed by performing a modified barium swallow test. If the aspiration is indirect (from acid reflux), then treatment is directed at this is indicated

Prevention

The evidence for the effectiveness of measures to prevent the development of asthma is weak. Ones which show some promise include: limiting smoke exposure both in utero and after delivery, breastfeeding, increased exposure to respiratory infection per the hygiene hypothesis (such as in those who attend daycare or are from large families).

Management

A specific, customized plan for proactively monitoring and managing symptoms should be created. Someone who has asthma should understand the importance of reducing exposure to allergens, testing to assess the severity of symptoms, and the usage of medications. The treatment plan should be written down and adjusted according to changes in symptoms. The most effective treatment for asthma is identifying triggers, such as cigarette smoke, pets, or aspirin, and eliminating exposure to them. If trigger avoidance is insufficient, medical treatment is recommended. Medical treatments used depends on the severity of illness and the frequency of symptoms. Specific medications for asthma are broadly classified into fast-acting and long-acting categories. Bronchodilators are recommended for short-term relief of symptoms. In those with occasional attacks, no other medication is needed. If mild persistent disease is present (more than two attacks a week), low-dose inhaled glucocorticoids or alternatively, an oral leukotriene antagonist or a mast cell stabilizer is recommended. For those who suffer daily attacks, a higher dose of inhaled glucocorticoid is used. In a severe asthma exacerbation, oral glucocorticoids are added to these treatments.

Lifestyle modification

Avoidance of triggers is a key component of improving control and preventing attacks. The most common triggers include: allergens, smoke (tobacco and other), air pollution, non-selective beta-blockers, and sulfite-containing foods.

Medications

Medications used to treat asthma are divided into two general classes: quick-relief medications used to treat acute symptoms; and long-term control medications used to prevent further exacerbation.

Salbutamol metered dose inhaler commonly used to treat asthma attacks.

Fast acting

Short acting beta$_2$-adrenoceptor agonists (SABA), such as salbutamol (*albuterol* USAN) are the first line treatment for asthma symptoms. Anticholinergic medications, such as ipratropium bromide provide addition benefit when used in combination with SABA in those with moderate or severe symptoms.

Anticholinergic bronchodilators can also be used if a person cannot tolerate a SABA. Older, less selective adrenergic agonists, such as inhaled epinephrine, have similar efficacy to SABAs. They are however not recommended due to concerns regarding excessive cardiac stimulation. Long term control

Fluticasone propionate metered dose inhaler commonly used for long term control.

Glucocorticoids are the most effective treatment available for long term control. Inhaled forms are usually used except in the case of severe persistent disease, in which oral steroids may be needed. Inhaled formulations may be used once or twice daily, depending on the severity of symptoms.

Long acting beta-adrenoceptor agonists (LABA) have at least a 12-hour effect. They are however not to be used without a steroid due to an increased risk of severe symptoms. In December 2008, members of the FDA's drug-safety office recommended withdrawing approval for these medications in children. Discussion is ongoing about their use in adults.

Leukotriene antagonists (such as zafirlukast) are an alternative to inhaled glucocorticoids, but are not preferred. They may also be used in addition to inhaled glucocorticoids but in this role are second line to LABA.

Mast cell stabilizers (such as cromolyn sodium) are another non-preferred alternative to glucocorticoids.

Delivery methods

Medications are typically provided as metered-dose inhalers (MDIs) in combination with an asthma spacer or as a dry powder inhaler. The spacer is a plastic cylinder that mixes the medication with air, making it easier to receive a full dose of the drug. A nebulizer may also be used. Nebulizers and spacers are equally effective in those with mild to moderate symptoms however insufficient evidence is available to determine whether or not a difference exist in that severe symptomatology.

Safety and adverse effects

Long-term use of glucocorticoids carries a significant potential for adverse effects. The incidence of cataracts is increased in people undergoing treatment for asthma with corticosteroids, due to altered regulation of lens epithelial cells.[1] The incidence of osteoporosis is also increased, due to changes in bone remodeling.

Other

When an asthma attack is unresponsive to usual medications, other options are available for emergency management.

Oxygen is used to alleviate hypoxia if saturations fall below 92%.

Magnesium sulfate intravenous treatment has been shown to provide a bronchodilation effect when used in addition to other treatment in severe acute asthma attacks.

Heliox, a mixture of helium and oxygen, may also be considered in severe unresponsive cases

Intravenous salbutamol is not supported by available evidence and is thus used only in extreme cases.

Methylxanthines (such as theophylline) were once widely used, but do not add significantly to the effects of inhaled beta-agonists

The dissociative anesthetic ketamine is theoretically useful

if intubation and mechanical ventilation is needed in people who are approaching respiratory arrest; however, there is no evidence from clinical trials to support this.

Complementary medicine

Many people with asthma, like those who suffer from other chronic disorders,

use alternative treatments; surveys show that roughly 50% of asthma patients use some form of unconventional therapy. There is little data to support the effectiveness of most of these therapies. Evidence is insufficient to support the usage of Vitamin C.

Acupuncture is not recommended for the treatment as there is insufficient evidence to support its use. Air ionizers show no evidence that they improve asthma symptoms or benefit lung function; this applied equally to positive and negative ion generators.

Dust mite control measures, including air filtration, chemicals to kill mites, vacuuming, mattress covers and others methods had no effect on asthma symptoms. However, a review of 30 studies found that "bedding encasement might be an effective asthma treatment under some conditions" (when the patient is highly allergic to dust mite and the intervention reduces the dust mite exposure level from high levels to low levels). Washing laundry/rugs in hot water was also found to improve control of allergens.

A study of "manual therapies" for asthma,

including osteopathic, chiropractic, physiotherapeutic and respiratory therapeuticmanoeuvres, found there is insufficient evidence to support their use in treating. The Buteyko breathing technique for controlling hyperventilation may result in a reduction in medications use however does not have any effect on lung function. Thus, an expert panel felt that evidence was insufficient to support its use.

Prognosis

The prognosis for asthma is good, especially for children with mild disease.[1] Of asthma diagnosed during childhood, 54% of cases will no longer carry the diagnosis after a decade the extent of permanent lung damage in people with asthma is unclear. Airway remodeling is observed, but it is unknown whether these represent harmful or beneficial changes.

Although conclusions from studies are mixed, most studies show that early treatment with glucocorticoids prevents or ameliorates decline in lung function as measured by several parameters. For those who continue to suffer from mild symptoms, corticosteroids can help most to live their lives with few disabilities. It is more likely to consider immediate medication of inhaled corticosteroids as soon as asthma attacks occur. According to studies conducted, patients with relatively mild asthma who have received inhaled corticosteroids within 12 months of their first asthma symptoms achieved good functional control of asthma after 10 years of individualized therapy as compared to patients who received this medication after 2 years (or more) from their first attacks Though they (delayed) also had good functional control of asthma, they were observed to exhibit slightly less optimal disease control and more signs of airway inflammation

Asthma mortality has decreased over the last few decades due to better recognition and improvement in care.

Respiratory failure

The term respiratory failure, in medicine, is used to describe inadequate gas exchange by the respiratory system, with the result that arterial oxygen and/or carbon dioxide levels cannot be maintained within their normal ranges. A drop in blood oxygenation is known as hypoxemia; a rise in arterial carbon dioxide levels is called hypercapnia. The normal reference values are: oxygen PaO_2 greater than 80 mmHg (11 kPa), and carbon dioxide $PaCO_2$ less than 45 mmHg (6.0 kPa). Classification into type I or type II relates to the absence or presence of hypercapnia respectively.

Types

Type 1

Type 1 respiratory failure is defined as hypoxemia without hypercapnia, and indeed the P_aCO_2 may be normal or low. It is typically caused by a ventilation/perfusion (V/Q) mismatch; the volume of air flowing in and out of the lungs is not matched with the flow of blood to the lungs. The basic defect in type 1 respiratory failure is failure of oxygenation characterized by:

P_aO_2

low (< 60 mmHg (8.0 kPa))

P_aCO_2

normal or low

$PA-aO2$

increased

This type of respiratory failure is caused by conditions that affect oxygenation such as:

Parenchymal disease (V/Q mismatch)

Diseases of vasculature and shunts: right-to-left shunt, pulmonary embolism

interstitial lung diseases: ARDS, pneumonia, emphysema.

Type 2

The basic defect in type 2 respiratory failure is characterized by:

P_aO_2

decreased

P_aCO_2

increased

$PA-aO2$

normal

pH

decreased

Type 2 respiratory failure is caused by increased airway resistance; both oxygen and carbon dioxide are affected. Defined as the buildup of carbon dioxide levels (P_aCO_2) that has been generated by the body. The underlying causes include:

Reduced breathing effort (in the fatigued patient)

A decrease in the area of the lung available for gas exchange (such as in emphysema).

Chest X-ray showing ARDS

Causes

    Pulmonary dysfunction

    Asthma

Emphysema
Chroni

CHAPTER TWENTY-SIX

GASTROENTERITIS

Gastroenteritis (also known as gastric flu, stomach flu, and stomach virus, although unrelated to influenza) is marked by severe inflammation of the gastrointestinal tract involving both the stomach and small intestine resulting in acute diarrhea and vomiting. It can be transferred by contact with contaminated food and water. The inflammation is caused most often by an infection from certain viruses or less often by bacteria,

their toxins (e.g. SEB), parasites, or an adverse reaction to something in the diet or medication.

At least 50% of cases of gastroenteritis resulting from foodborne illness are caused by norovirus. Another 20% of cases, and the majority of severe cases in children, are due to rotavirus. Other significant viral agents include adenovirus and astrovirus.

Different species of bacteria can cause gastroenteritis, including *Salmonella, Shigella,Staphylococcus, Campylobacter*

jejuni, Clostridium, Escherichia coli, Yersinia, Vibrio cholerae, and others. Some sources of the infection are improperly prepared food, reheated meat dishes, seafood, dairy, and bakery products. Each organism causes slightly different symptoms but all result in diarrhea. Colitis, inflammation of the large intestine, may also be present.

Risk factors include consumption of improperly prepared foods or contaminated water and travel or residence in areas of poor sanitation. It is also common for river swimmers to become infected during times of rain as a result of contaminated runoff water.

Classification

Infectious gastroenteritis is caused by a wide variety of bacteria and viruses. It is important to consider infectious gastroenteritis as a diagnosis per exclusionism. A few loose stools and vomiting may be the result of systemic infection such as pneumonia, septicemia, urinary tract infection and even meningitis. Surgical conditions such

as appendicitis, intussusception and, rarely, even Hirschsprung's disease may mislead the clinician. Endocrine disorders (e.g. thyrotoxicosis and Addison's disease) are disorders that can cause diarrhea. Also, pancreatic insufficiency, short bowel syndrome, Whipple's disease, coeliac disease, and laxative abuse should be excluded as possibilities.[4]

Bacterial gastroenteritis

For a list of bacteria causing gastroenteritis, see above. Pseudomembranous colitis is an important cause of diarrhea in patients often recently treated with broad-spectrum antibiotics. Traveler's diarrhea is usually a type of bacterial gastroenteritis.

If gastroenteritis in a child is severe enough to require admission to a hospital, then it is important to distinguish between bacterial and viral infections. Bacteria

like, *Shigella* and *Campylobacter*, and parasites like *Giardia* can be treated with antibiotics.

Viral gastroenteritis

Viruses causing gastroenteritis include rotavirus, norovirus, adenovirus and astrovirus. Viruses do not respond to antibiotics and infected children usually make a full recovery after a few days.[5]Children admitted to hospital with gastroenteritis routinely are tested for rotavirus A to gather surveillance data relevant to the epidemiological effects of rotavirus vaccination programs. These children are routinely tested also for norovirus, which is extraordinarily infectious and requires special isolation procedures to avoid transmission to other patients. Other methods, electron microscopy and polyacrylamide gel electrophoresis, are used in research laboratories.

Symptoms and signs

Gastroenteritis often involves stomach pain or spasms, diarrhea and/or vomiting, with noninflammatory infection of the upper small bowel, or inflammatory infections of the colon.

The condition is usually of acute onset, normally lasting 1–6 days, and is self-limiting.

Nausea and vomiting
Dehydration
Diarrhea
Loss of appetite
Fever
Headaches
Abnormal flatulence
Abdominal pain
Abdominal cramps
Bloody stools (dysentery - suggesting infection by
amoeba, *Campylobacter*, *Salmonella*, *Shigella* or some pathogenic strains of *Escherichia coli*)
Fainting and Weakness
Heartburn

The main contributing factors include poor feeding in infants. Diarrhea is common, and may be followed by vomiting. Viral diarrhea usually causes frequent watery stools, whereas blood stained diarrhea may be indicative of bacterial colitis. In some cases, even when the stomach is empty, bile can be vomited up.

A child with gastroenteritis may be lethargic, suffer lack of sleep, run a low fever, have signs of dehydration (which include dry mucous membranes), tachycardia, reduced skin turgor, skin color discoloration, sunken fontanelles, sunken eyeballs, darkened eye circles, glassy eyes, poor perfusion and ultimately shock.

Diagnosis

Gastroenteritis is diagnosed based on symptoms, a complete medical history and a physical examination. An accurate medical history may provide valuable information on the existence or inexistence of similar symptoms in other members of the patient's family or friends. The duration, frequency, and description of the patient's bowel movements and if they experience vomiting are also relevant and these questions are usually asked by a physician during the examination.

No specific diagnostic tests are required in most patients with simple gastroenteritis. If symptoms including fever, bloody stool and diarrhea persist for two weeks or more, examination of stool for Clostridium difficile may be advisable along with cultures for bacteria including Salmonella, Shigella, Campylobacter and enterotoxin Escherichia coli. Microscopy for parasites, ova and cysts may also be helpful

A complete medical history may be helpful in diagnosing gastroenteritis. A complete and accurate medical history of the patient includes information on travel history, exposure to poisons or other irritants, diet change, food preparation habits or storage and

medications. Patients who travel may be exposed to E. Coli infections or parasite infections contacted from beverages or food. Swimming in contaminated water or drinking from suspicious fresh water such as mountain streams or wells may indicate infection from *Giardia* - an organism found in water that causes diarrhea.

Food poisoning must be considered in cases when the patient was exposed to undercooked or improperly stored food. Depending on the type of bacteria that is causing the condition, the reactions appear in 2 to 72 hours. Detecting the specific infectious agent is required in order to establish a proper diagnosis and an effective treatment plan.

The doctor may want to find whether the patient has been using broad-spectrum or multiple antibiotics in their recent past. If so, they could be the cause of an irritation of the gastrointestinal tract.

During the physical examination, the doctor will look for other possible causes of the infection. Conditions such

as appendicitis, gallbladder disease, pancreatitis or diverticulitis may cause similar symptoms but a physical examination will reveal a specific tenderness in the abdomen which is not present in gastroenteritis.

Diagnosing gastroenteritis is mainly an exclusion procedure. Therefore, in rare cases when the symptoms are not enough to diagnose gastroenteritis, several tests may be performed in order to rule out other gastrointestinal disorders. These include rectal examinations, complete blood count, electrolytes and kidney function tests. However, when

the symptoms are conclusive, no tests apart from the stool tests are required to correctly diagnose gastroenteritis especially if the patient has traveled to at-risk areas.

Percentage of rotavirus tests with positive results, by surveillance week, United States, July 2000--June 2009.

Prevention

Since 2000, the implementation of a rotavirus vaccine has decreased the number of cases of diarrhea due to rotavirus in the United States.

Gastroenteritis may be prevented through immunization. The U.S. Food and Drug Administration approved in 2006 a rotavirus vaccine called Rotate that may be given to infants aged 6 to 32 weeks to prevent getting infected with viral gastroenteritis. The vaccines may however have side effects that are similar to the mild flu symptoms.

Different types of vaccinations are available for Salmonella typhi and Vibrio cholera and which may be administered to people who intend traveling in at-risk areas. However, the vaccines that are currently available are effective only on rotaviral gastroenteritis.

Doctors recommend that food be properly cooked and stored to prevent gastroenteritis. Avoid suspect food or drink. Thoroughly wash both hands before eating and after using the bathroom or changing diapers. Viral gastroenteritis is a highly contagious disease and thus avoiding crowded spaces such as markets, theaters or shopping centers may also help in preventing infection for those who have weak resistance. Bleaching soiled laundry and household surfaces may help prevent spreading bacteria.

Management

Gastroenteritis is usually an acute and self-limited disease that does not require pharmacological therapy. The objective of treatment is to replace

lost fluids and electrolytes. Oral rehydration is the preferred method of replacing these losses in children with mild to moderate

dehydration. Metoclopramide and ondansetron however may be helpful in children.

Rehydration

The primary treatment of gastroenteritis in both children and adults is rehydration, i.e., replenishment of water and electrolytes lost in the stools. This is preferably achieved by giving the person oral rehydration therapy (ORT) although intravenous delivery may be required if a decreased level of consciousness or an ileus is present. Complex- carbohydrate-based oral rehydration therapy such as those made from wheat or rice may be superior to simple sugar-based ORS.

Sugary drinks such as soft drinks and fruit juice are not recommended for gastroenteritis in children under 5 years of age as they may make the diarrhea worse. Plain water may be used if specific ORS are unavailable or not palatable.

Diet

It is recommended that breastfed infants continue to be nursed on demand and that formula-fed infants should continue their usual formula immediately after rehydration with oral rehydration solutions. Lactose-free or lactose-reduced formulas usually are not necessary.

Children receiving semisolid or solid foods should continue to receive their usual diet during episodes of diarrhea. Foods high in simple sugars should be avoided because the osmotic load might worsen diarrhea; therefore, substantial amounts of soft drinks, juice, and other high simple sugar foods should be avoided. The practice of withholding food is not recommended and immediate normal feeding is encouraged The BRAT diet (bananas, rice, applesauce, toast and tea) is no longer recommended, as it contains insufficient nutrients and has no benefit over normal feeding.

Medications

Antiemetics

Antiemetic drugs may be helpful for vomiting in children. Ondansetron has some utility with a single dose associated with less need for intravenous fluids, fewer hospitalizations, and decreased vomiting. Metoclopramide also might be helpful. However, there was an increased number of children who returned and were subsequently admitted in those treated with ondansetron. The intravenous preparation of ondansetron may be given orally.

Antibiotics

Antibiotics are not usually used for gastroenteritis, although they are sometimes used if symptoms are severe (such as dysentery) or a susceptible bacterial cause is isolated or suspected. If antibiotics are decided on, a fluoroquinolone or macrolide is often used.

Pseudomembranous colitis, usually caused by antibiotics use, is managed by discontinuing the causative agent and treating with either metronidazole or vancomycin.

Antimotility agents

Antimotility drugs have a theoretical risk of causing complications; clinical experience, however, has shown this to be unlikely. They are thus discouraged in people with bloody diarrhea or diarrhea complicated by a fever.]Loperamide, an opioid analogue, is commonly used for the symptomatic treatment of diarrhea. Loperamide is not recommended in children as it may cross the immature blood brain barrier and cause toxicity. Bismuth subsalicylate (BSS), an insoluble complex of trivalent bismuth and salicylate, can be used in mild-moderate cases.

Antispasmodics

Butyl scopolamine (Buscopan) is useful in treating crampy abdominal pain.

Alternative medicine

Probiotics

Some probiotics have been shown to be beneficial in preventing and treating various forms of gastroenteritis. They reduce both the duration of illness and the frequency of

stools. Fermented milk products (such as yogurt) also reduce the duration of symptoms.[35]

Zinc

The World Health Organization recommends that infants and children receive a dietary supplement of zinc for up to two weeks after onset of gastroenteritis. A 2009 trial however did not find any benefit from supplementation.

Complications

Dehydration is a common complication of diarrhea. It can be made worse with the withholding fluids or the administration of juice / soft drinks. Malabsorption of lactose, the principal sugar in milk, may occur. Though it may increase the diarrhea, however, mothers should continue breastfeeding.

History

Before the 20th century, the term "gastroenteritis" was not commonly used. What would now be diagnosed as gastroenteritis may have instead been diagnosed more*specifically* as typhoid fever or "cholera morbus", among

others, or *less specifically* as "griping of the guts", "surfeit", "flux", "colic", "bowel complaint", or any one of a number of
other archaic names for acute diarrhea. Historians, genealogists, and other researchers should keep in mind that gastroenteritis was not considered a discrete diagnosis until fairly recently.

U.S. President Zachary Taylor died of "cholera morbus", equivalent to a diagnosis of gastroenteritis, on July 9, 1850.

CHAPTER TWENTY-SEVEN

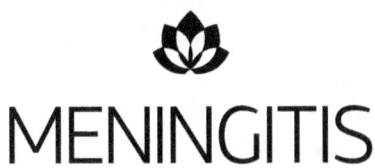

MENINGITIS

Meningitis is inflammation of the protective membranes the brain and spinal cord, known collectively as the meninges. The inflammation may be caused by infection with viruses, bacteria, or other microorganisms covering, and less commonly by

certain drugs Meningitis can be life-threatening because of the inflammation's proximity to the brain and spinal cord; therefore, the condition is classified as a medical emergency.[1][3]

The most common symptoms of meningitis are headache and neck stiffness associated with fever, confusion or altered consciousness, vomiting, and an inability to tolerate light

(photophobia) or loud noises (phonophobia). Sometimes, especially in small children, only nonspecific symptoms may be present, such as irritability and drowsiness. If a rash is present, it may indicate a particular cause of meningitis; for instance, meningitis caused by meningococcal bacteria may be accompanied by a characteristic rash.

A lumbar puncture may be used to diagnose or exclude meningitis. This involves inserting a needle into the spinal canal to extract a sample of cerebrospinal fluid (CSF), the fluid that envelops the brain and spinal cord. The CSF is then examined in a medical laboratory. The usual treatment for meningitis is the prompt application of antibiotics and sometimes antiviral drugs. In some situations, corticosteroid drugs can also be used to prevent complications from overactive inflammation. Meningitis can lead to serious long-term consequences such as deafness, epilepsy, hydrocephalus and cognitive deficits, especially if not treated quickly. Some forms of meningitis (such as those associated

with meningococci, *Hemophilus influenzae* type B, pneumococci or mumps virus infections) may be prevented by immunization.

Signs and symptoms
  Clinical features

Neck stiffness, Texas Meningitis Epidemic of 1911–12.
  In adults, a severe headache is the most common symptom of meningitis – occurring in almost 90% of cases of bacterial meningitis, followed by nuchal rigidity (inability to flex the neck forward passively due to increased neck muscle tone and stiffness). The classic triad of diagnostic signs consists of nuchal rigidity, sudden high fever, and altered mental status; however, all three features are present in only 44–46% of all cases of bacterial meningitis. If none of the three signs is present, meningitis is extremely unlikely. Other signs commonly
  associated with meningitis include photophobia (intolerance to bright light)
  and phonophobia (intolerance to loud noises). Small children often do not exhibit the aforementioned symptoms, and may only be irritable and look unwell. In infants up to
  6 months of age, bulging of the fontanelle (the soft spot on top of a baby's head) may be present. Other features that might distinguish meningitis from less severe illnesses in young children are leg pain, cold extremities, and an abnormal skin color.
  Nuchal rigidity occurs in 70% of adult cases of bacterial meningitis. Other signs

of meningism include the presence of positive Kernig's sign or Brudzinski's sign. Kernig's sign is assessed with the patient lying supine, with the hip and knee flexed to 90 degrees. In a patient with a positive Kernig's sign, pain limits passive extension of the knee. A positive Brudzinski's sign occurs when flexion of the neck causes involuntary flexion of the knee and hip. Although Kernig's and Brudzinski's signs are both commonly used to screen for meningitis, the sensitivity of these tests is limited. They do, however, have very

good specificity for meningitis: the signs rarely occurs in other diseases. Another test, known as the "jolt accentuation maneuver" helps determine whether meningitis is present in patients reporting fever and headache. The patient is told to rapidly rotate his or her head horizontally; if this does not make the headache worse, meningitis is unlikely.

Meningitis caused by the bacterium *Neisseria meningitidis* (known as "meningococcal meningitis") can be differentiated from meningitis with other causes by a rapidly spreading petechial rash which may precede other symptoms. The rash consists of

numerous small, irregular purple or red spots ("petechiae") on the trunk, lower extremities, mucous membranes, conjunctiva, and (occasionally) the palms of the hands or soles of the feet. The rash is typically non-blanching: the redness does not disappear when pressed with a finger or a glass tumbler. Although this rash is not necessarily present in meningococcal meningitis, it is relatively specific for the disease; it does, however, occasionally occur in meningitis due to other bacteria. Other clues as to the nature of the cause of meningitis may be the skin signs of hand, foot and mouth disease and genital herpes, both of which are associated with various forms of viral meningitis.

Early complications

A severe case of meningococcal meningitis in which the petechial rash progressed to gangreneand requiredamputationof all limbs.

People with meningitis may develop additional problems in the early stages of their illness. These may require specific treatment, and sometimes indicate severe illness or worse prognosis. The infection may trigger sepsis, a systemic inflammatory response syndrome of falling blood pressure, fast heart rate, high or abnormally low temperature and rapid breathing. Very low blood pressure may occur early, especially but not exclusively in meningococcal illness; this may lead to insufficient blood supply to other

organs. Disseminated intravascular coagulation, the excessive activation of blood clotting, may cause both the obstruction of blood flow to organs and a paradoxical increase of bleeding risk. In meningococcal disease, gangrene of limbs can occur. Severe meningococcal and pneumococcal infections may result in hemorrhaging of the adrenal glands, leading to Waterhouse-Frederiksen syndrome, which is often lethal. The brain tissue may swell, with increasing pressure inside the skull and a risk of swollen brain tissue causing herniation. This may be noticed by a decreasing level of consciousness, loss of the pupillary light reflex, and abnormal posturing.

Inflammation of the brain tissue may also obstruct the normal flow of CSF around the brain (hydrocephalus). Seizures may occur for various reasons; in children, seizures are common in the early stages of meningitis (30% of cases) and do not necessarily indicate an underlying cause. Seizures may result from increased pressure and from areas of inflammation in the brain tissue. Focal seizures (seizures that involve one limb or part of the body), persistent seizures, late-onset seizures and those that are difficult to control with medication are indicators of a poorer long-term outcome.

The inflammation of the meninges may lead to abnormalities of the cranial nerves, a group of nerves arising from the brain stem that supply the head and neck area and control eye movement, facial muscles and hearing, among other functions. Visual symptoms

and hearing loss may persist after an episode of meningitis (see below). Inflammation of the

brain (encephalitis) or its blood vessels (cerebral vasculitis), as well as the formation

of blood clots in the veins (cerebral venous thrombosis), may all lead to weakness, loss of sensation, or abnormal movement or function of the part of the body supplied by the affected area in the brain.

Causes

Meningitis is usually caused by infection from viruses or micro-organisms. Most cases are due to infection with viruses, with bacteria, fungi, and parasites being the next most common causes It may also result from various non-infectious causes.

Bacterial

The types of bacteria that because bacterial meningitis vary by age group. In premature babies and newborns up to three months old, common causes are *group B*

streptococci (subtypes III which normally inhabit the vagina and are mainly a cause during the first week of life) and those that normally inhabit the digestive tract such as *Escherichia coli* (carrying K1 antigen). *Listeria monocytogenes* (serotype Vibe) may affect the newborn and occurs in epidemics. Older children are more commonly affected by *Neisseria meningitidis* (meningococcus), *Streptococcus pneumoniae* (serotypes 6, 9, 14, 18 and 23) and those under five by *Hemophilus influenzae* type B (in countries that do not offer vaccination, see below). In adults, *N. meningitidis* and *S. pneumoniae* together cause 80% of all cases of bacterial meningitis, with increased risk of *L. monocytogenes* in those over 50 years old. Since the pneumococcal vaccine was introduced, however, rates of pneumococcal meningitis have declined in children and adults.

Recent trauma to the skull gives bacteria in the nasal cavity the potential to enter the meningeal space. Similarly, individuals with a cerebral shunt or related device (such as an extra ventricular drain or Ommaya reservoir) are at increased risk of infection through those devices. In these cases, infections with staphylococci are more likely, as well as

infections by pseudomonas and other Gram-negative bacilli. The same pathogens are also more common in those with an impaired immune system.in a small proportion of people, an infection in the head and neck area, such as otitis media or mastoiditis, can lead to meningitis. Recipients of cochlear implants for hearing loss are at an increased risk of pneumococcal meningitis.

Tuberculous meningitis, meningitis due to infection with *Mycobacterium tuberculosis*, is more common in those from countries where tuberculosis is common, but is also encountered in those with immune problems, such as AIDS. Recurrent bacterial meningitis

may be caused by persisting anatomical defects, either congenital or acquired, or by disorders of the immune system. Anatomical defects allow continuity between the external environment and the nervous system. The most common cause of recurrent meningitis

is skull fracture, particularly fractures that affect the base of the skull or extend towards the sinuses and petrous pyramids. A literature review of 363 reported cases of recurrent

meningitis showed that 59% of cases are due to such anatomical abnormalities, 36% due to immune deficiencies (such as complement deficiency, which predisposes especially to recurrent meningococcal meningitis), and 5% due to ongoing infections in areas adjacent to the meninges.

Aseptic

The term *aseptic meningitis* refers loosely to all cases of meningitis in which no bacterial infection can be demonstrated. This is usually due to viruses, but it may be due to bacterial infection that has already been partially treated, with disappearance of the bacteria from the meninges, or by infection in a space adjacent to the meninges

(e.g. sinusitis). Endocarditis (infection of the heart valves with spread of small clusters of bacteria through the bloodstream) may cause aseptic meningitis. Aseptic meningitis may also result from infection with spirochetes, a type of bacteria that includes *Treponema pallidum* (the cause of syphilis) and *Borrelia burgdorferi* (known for causing Lyme disease). Meningitis may be encountered in cerebral malaria (malaria infecting the brain). Fungal meningitis, e.g. due to *Cryptococcus neoformans*, is typically seen in people with immune deficiency such as AIDS. Amoebic meningitis, meningitis due to infection with amoebae such as *Naegleria fowleri*, is contracted from freshwater sources.[2]

Viral

Viruses that can cause meningitis include enteroviruses, herpes simplex virus type 2 (and less commonly type 1), varicella zoster virus (known for

causing chickenpox and shingles), mumps virus, HIV, and LCMV.[9]

Parasitic

A parasitic cause is often assumed when there is a predominance of eosinophils (a type of white blood cell) in the CSF. The most common parasites implicated are *Angiostrongyliasis cantonensis*, *Gnathostoma spinigerum*, *Schistosoma*, as well as the conditions cysticercosis, toxocariasis, Baylis ascariasis, paragonimiasis, and a number of rarer infections and noninfective conditions.[15]

Non-infectious

Meningitis may occur as the result of several non-infectious causes: spread of cancer to the meninges (*malignant meningitis*) and certain drugs (mainly non-steroidal anti-inflammatory drugs, antibiotics and intravenous immunoglobulins). It may also be caused by several inflammatory conditions such as sarcoidosis (which is then called neurosarcoidosis), connective tissue disorders such as systemic lupus erythematosus, and certain forms

of vasculitis (inflammatory conditions of the blood vessel wall) such as Bechet's disease. Epidermoid cysts and dermoid cysts may cause meningitis by releasing irritant matter into the subarachnoid space. Mollaret's meningitis is a syndrome of recurring episodes of aseptic meningitis; it is thought to be caused by herpes simplex virus type 2.

Rarely, migraine may cause meningitis, but this diagnosis is usually only made when other causes have been eliminated.

Mechanism

The meninges comprise three membranes that, together with the cerebrospinal fluid, enclose and protect the brain and spinal cord (the central nervous system). The pia mater is a very delicate impermeable membrane that firmly adheres to the surface of the brain, following all the minor contours. The arachnoid mater (so named because of its spider-web-like appearance) is a loosely fitting sac on top of the pia mater. The subarachnoid

space separates the arachnoid and pia mater membranes, and is filled with cerebrospinal fluid. The outermost membrane, the dura mater, is a thick durable membrane, which is attached to both the arachnoid membrane and the skull.

In bacterial meningitis, bacteria reach the meninges by one of two main routes: through the bloodstream or through direct contact between the meninges and either the nasal cavity or the skin. In most cases, meningitis follows invasion of the bloodstream by organisms that live upon mucous surfaces such as the nasal cavity. This is often in turn preceded by viral infections, which break down the normal barrier provided by the mucous surfaces. Once bacteria have entered the bloodstream, they enter the subarachnoid space in places where the blood-brain barrier is vulnerable—such as the choroid plexus. Meningitis occurs in 25% of newborns with bloodstream infections due to group B streptococci; this phenomenon is less common in adults. Direct contamination of the cerebrospinal fluid may arise from indwelling devices, skull fractures, or infections of the nasopharynx or the nasal sinuses that have formed a tract with the subarachnoid space (see above); occasionally, congenital defects of the dura mater can be identified.

The large-scale inflammation that occurs in the subarachnoid space during meningitis is not a direct result of bacterial infection but can rather largely be attributed to the response of

the immune system to the entrance of bacteria into the central nervous system. When components of the bacterial cell membrane are identified by the immune cells of the brain (astrocytes and microglia), they respond by releasing large amounts of cytokines, hormone-like mediators that recruit other immune cells and stimulate other tissues to participate in an immune response. The blood-brain barrier becomes more permeable, leading

to "vasogenic" cerebral edema (swelling of the brain due to fluid leakage from blood vessels). Large numbers of white blood cells enter the CSF, causing inflammation of the meninges, and leading to "interstitial" edema (swelling due to fluid between the cells). In addition, the walls of the blood vessels themselves become inflamed (cerebral vasculitis), which leads to a decreased blood flow and a third type of edema, "cytotoxic" edema. The three forms of cerebral edema all lead to an increased intracranial pressure; together with the lowered blood pressure often encountered in acute infection, this means that it is harder for blood to enter the brain, and brain cells are deprived of oxygen and

undergo apoptosis (automated cell death).

It is recognized that administration of antibiotics may initially worsen the process outlined above, by increasing the amount of bacterial cell membrane products released through the destruction of bacteria. Particular treatments, such as the use of corticosteroids, are aimed at dampening the immune system's response to this phenomenon.

Diagnosis

CSF findings in different forms of meningitis[18]

Type of meningitis

Glucose

Protein

Cells

Acute bacterial

low

high

PMNs,

often > 300/mm³

Acute viral

normal

normal or high

mononuclear,

< 300/mm³

Tuberculous

low

high

mononuclear and PMNs, < 300/mm³

Fungal

low

high

< 300/mm³

Malignant

low

high

usually mononuclear

Blood tests and imaging

In someone suspected of having meningitis, blood tests are performed for markers of inflammation (e.g. C-reactive protein, complete blood count), as well as blood cultures. The most important test in identifying or ruling out meningitis is analysis of the cerebrospinal fluid through lumbar puncture (LP, spinal tap). However, lumbar puncture is contraindicated if there is a mass in the brain (tumor or abscess) or the intracranial pressure (ICP) is elevated, as it may lead to brain herniation. If someone is at risk for either a mass or raised ICP (recent head injury, a known immune system problem, localizing neurological signs, or evidence on examination of a raised ICP), a CT ormyrid scan is recommended prior to the lumbar puncture. This applies in 45% of all adult cases. If a CT or MRI is required before LP, or if LP proves difficult, professional guidelines suggest that antibiotics should be administered first to prevent delay in treatment, especially if this may be longer than

30 minutes. Often, CT or MRI scans are performed at a later stage to assess for complications of meningitis.

In severe forms of meningitis, monitoring of blood electrolytes may be important; for example, hyponatremia is common in bacterial meningitis, due to a combination of factors including dehydration, the inappropriate excretion of the antidiuretic hormone (SIADH), or overly aggressive intravenous fluid administration.

Lumbar puncture

A lumbar puncture is done by positioning the patient, usually lying on the side,

applying local anesthetic, and inserting a needle into the Dural sac (a sac around the spinal cord) to collect cerebrospinal fluid (CSF). When this has been achieved, the "opening pressure" of the CSF is measured using a manometer. The pressure is normally between 6 and 18 cm water (cmH_2O in bacterial meningitis the pressure is typically elevated. The initial appearance of the fluid may prove an indication of the nature of the infection: cloudy CSF indicates higher levels of protein, white and red blood cells and/or bacteria, and therefore may suggest bacterial meningitis.

Gram stain of meningococci from a culture showing Gram negative (pink) bacteria, often in pairs

The CSF sample is examined for presence and types of white blood cells, red blood cells, protein content and glucose level. Gram staining of the sample may demonstrate bacteria in bacterial meningitis, but absence of bacteria does not exclude bacterial meningitis as they are only seen in 60% of cases; this figure is reduced by a further 20% if antibiotics were administered before the sample was taken, and Gram staining is also less reliable in particular infections such as listeriosis. Microbiological culture of the sample is more sensitive (it identifies the organism in 70–85% of cases) but results can take up to 48 hours to become available. The type of white blood cell predominantly present (see table) indicates whether meningitis is bacterial (usually neutrophil-predominant) or viral (usually lymphocyte-predominant), although in the beginning of the disease this is not always a reliable indicator. Less commonly, eosinophils predominate, suggesting parasitic or fungal etiology, among others. The concentration of glucose in CSF is normally above 40% that in blood. In bacterial meningitis it is typically lower; the CSF glucose level is

therefore, divided by the blood glucose (CSF glucose to serum glucose ratio). A ratio ≤0.4 is

indicative of bacterial meningitis; in the newborn, glucose levels in CSF are normally higher, and a ratio below 0.6 (60%) is therefore considered abnormal. High levels of lactate in CSF indicate a higher likelihood of bacterial meningitis, as does a higher white blood cell count.

Various more specialized tests may be used to distinguish between various types of meningitis. A latex agglutination test may be positive in meningitis caused by *Streptococcus pneumoniae*, *Neisseria meningitidis*, *Hemophilus influenzae*, *Escherichia coli* and *group B streptococci*; its routine use is not encouraged as it rarely leads to changes in treatment, but it may be used if other tests are not diagnostic. Similarly, the limulus lysate test may be positive in meningitis caused by Gram-negative bacteria, but it is of limited use unless other tests have been unhelpful. Polymerase chain reaction (PCR) is a technique used to amplify small traces of bacterial DNA in order to detect the presence of bacterial or viral DNA in cerebrospinal fluid; it is a highly sensitive and specific test since only trace amounts of the

infecting agent's DNA is required. It may identify bacteria in bacterial meningitis and may assist in distinguishing the various causes of viral meningitis (enterovirus, herpes simplex virus 2 and mumps in those not vaccinated for this). Serology (identification of antibodies to viruses) may be useful in viral meningitis. If tuberculous meningitis is suspected, the sample is processed for Ziehl-Neelsen stain, which has a low sensitivity, and tuberculosis culture, which takes a long time to process; PCR is being used increasingly. Diagnosis of cryptococcal meningitis can be made at low cost using an India ink stain of the CSF; however, testing for cryptococcal antigen in blood or CSF is more sensitive, particularly in persons with AIDS.

A diagnostic and therapeutic conundrum is the "partially treated meningitis", where there are meningitis symptoms after receiving antibiotics (such as for presumptive sinusitis).

When this happens, CSF findings may resemble those of viral meningitis, but antibiotic treatment may need to be continued until there is definitive positive evidence of a viral cause (e.g. a positive enterovirus PCR).

Histopathology of bacterial meningitis: autopsy case of a patient with pneumococcal meningitis showing inflammatory infiltrates of the pia mater consisting of neutrophil granulocytes (inset, higher magnification).

Postmortem

Meningitis can be diagnosed after death has occurred. The findings from a post mortem are usually a widespread inflammation of the pia mater and arachnoid layers of the meninges covering the brain and spinal cord. Neutrophil granulocytes tend to have migrated to the cerebrospinal fluid and the base of the brain, along with cranial nerves and the spinal cord, may be surrounded with pus—as may the meningeal vessels.

Prevention

Behavioral

Bacterial and viral meningitis are contagious. Neither are as contagious as the common cold or flu. Both can be transmitted through droplets of respiratory secretions during close contact such as kissing, sneezing or coughing on someone, but cannot be spread by only breathing the air where a person with meningitis has been. Viral meningitis is typically caused by Enteroviruses, and is most commonly spread through fecal contamination. By changing behavior to prevent the causes of transmission, infection by viruses and bacteria can be prevented.

Pharmaceutical

For some causes of meningitis, prophylaxis can be provided in the long term with vaccine, or in the short term with antibiotics.

Since the 1980s, many countries have included immunization against *Hemophilus influenzae* type B in their routine childhood vaccination schemes. This has practically eliminated this pathogen as a cause of meningitis in young children in those countries. In the countries where the disease burden is highest, however, the vaccine is still too expensive. Similarly, immunization against mumps has led to a sharp fall in the number of cases of mumps meningitis, which prior to vaccination occurred in 15% of all cases of mumps.

Meningococcus vaccines exist against groups A, C, W135 and Y. In countries where the vaccine for meningococcus group C was introduced, cases caused by this pathogen have decreased substantially. A quadrivalent vaccine now exists, which combines all four vaccines. Immunization with the ACW135Y vaccine against four strains is now a visa requirement for taking part in the Hajj.[1]Development of a vaccine against group B meningococci has proved much more difficult, as its surface proteins (which would normally be used to make a vaccine) only elicit a weak response from the immune system, or cross- react with normal human proteins. Still, some countries (New

Zealand, Cuba, Norway and Chile) have developed vaccines against local strains of group B meningococci; some have shown good results and are used in local immunization schedules. In Africa, the current approach for prevention and control of meningococcal epidemics is based on early detection of the disease and emergency reactive mass vaccination of the at-risk population with bivalent A/C or trivalent A/C/W135 polysaccharide vaccines.

Routine vaccination against *Streptococcus pneumoniae* with the pneumococcal conjugate vaccine (PCV), which is active against seven common serotypes of this pathogen, significantly reduces the incidence of pneumococcal meningitis. The pneumococcal

polysaccharide vaccine, which covers 23 strains, is only administered in certain groups (e.g. those who have had a splenectomy, the surgical removal of the spleen); it does not elicit a significant immune response in all recipients, e.g. small children.

Childhood vaccination with Bacillus Calmette-Guerin has been reported to significantly reduce the rate of tuberculous meningitis, but its waning effectiveness in adulthood has prompted a search for a better vaccine.

Short-term antibiotic prophylaxis is also a method of prevention, particularly of meningococcal meningitis. In cases of meningococcal meningitis, prophylactic treatment of close contacts with antibiotics (e.g. rifampicin, ciprofloxacin or ceftriaxone) can reduce their risk of contracting the condition, but does not protect against future infections.

Treatment
Initial treatment

Meningitis is potentially life-threatening and has a high mortality rate if untreated; delay in treatment has been associated with a poorer outcome. Thus, treatment with wide-spectrum antibiotics should not be delayed while confirmatory tests are being conducted. If meningococcal disease is suspected in primary care, guidelines recommend

that benzylpenicillin be administered before transfer to hospital. Intravenous fluids should be administered if hypotension (low blood pressure) or shock are present.[21]Given that meningitis can cause a number of early severe complications, regular medical review is recommended to identify these complications early as well as admission to an intensive care unit if deemed necessary.

Mechanical ventilation may be needed if the level of consciousness is very low, or if there is evidence of respiratory failure. If there are signs of raised intracranial pressure, measures to monitor the pressure may be taken; this would allow the optimization of the cerebral perfusion pressure and various treatments to decrease the intracranial pressure with medication (e.g. mannitol). Seizures are treated with anticonvulsants. Hydrocephalus (obstructed flow of CSF) may require insertion of a temporary or long-term drainage device, such as a cerebral shunt.

Bacterial meningitis

Structural formula of ceftriaxone, one of the third-generation cephalosporin antibiotics recommended for the initial treatment of bacterial meningitis.

Antibiotics

Empiric antibiotics (treatment without exact diagnosis) must be started immediately, even before the results of the lumbar puncture and CSF analysis are known. The choice of initial treatment depends largely on the kind of bacteria that cause meningitis in a particular place. For instance, in the United Kingdom empirical treatment consists of a third- generationcefalosporin such as cefotaxime or ceftriaxone. In the USA, where resistance to cephalosporins is increasingly found in streptococci, addition of vancomycin to the initial treatment is recommended. Empirical therapy may be chosen on the basis of the age of the patient, whether the infection was preceded by head injury, whether the patient has undergone neurosurgery and whether or not a cerebral shunt is present. For instance, in young children and those over 50 years of age, as well as those who are immunocompromised, addition of ampicillin is recommended to cover *Listeria monocytogenes*. Once the Gram stain results become available, and the broad type of bacterial cause is known, it may be possible to change the antibiotics to those likely to deal with the presumed group of pathogens.

The results of the CSF culture generally take longer to become available (24–48 hours). Once they do, empiric therapy may be switched to specific antibiotic therapy targeted to the specific causative organism and its sensitivities to antibiotics. For an antibiotic to be effective in meningitis, it must not only be active against the pathogenic bacterium, but also reach the meninges in adequate quantities; some antibiotics have inadequate penetrance and therefore have little use in meningitis. Most of the antibiotics used in meningitis have not been tested directly on meningitis patients in clinical trials. Rather, the relevant knowledge has mostly derived from laboratory studies in rabbits. Tuberculous meningitis requires prolonged treatment with antibiotics. While tuberculosis of the lungs is typically treated for six months, those with tuberculous meningitis are typically treated for a year or

longer. In tuberculous meningitis there is a strong evidence base for treatment with corticosteroids, although this evidence is restricted to those without AIDS.

Steroids

Adjuvant treatment with corticosteroids (usually dexamethasone) has been shown in some studies to reduce rates of mortality, severe hearing loss and neurological damage in adolescents and adults from high income countries which have low rates of HIV. The likely mechanism is suppression of overactive inflammation. Professional guidelines therefore recommend the commencement of dexamethasone or a similar corticosteroid just before the first dose of antibiotics is given, and continued for four days. Given that most of the benefit of the treatment is confined to those with pneumococcal meningitis, some guidelines suggest that dexamethasone be discontinued if another cause for meningitis is identified.

Adjuvant corticosteroids have a different role in children than in adults. Though the benefit of corticosteroids has been demonstrated in adults as well as in children from high-income countries, their use in children from low-income countries is not supported by evidence; the reason for this discrepancy is not clear. Even in high-income countries, the benefit of corticosteroids is only seen when they are given prior to the first dose of antibiotics, and is greatest in cases of *H. influenzae* meningitis, the incidence of which has decreased dramatically since the introduction of the Hib vaccine. Thus, corticosteroids are recommended in the treatment of pediatric meningitis if the cause is *H. influenzae* and only if given prior to the first dose of antibiotics, whereas other uses are controversial.

A 2010 analysis of previous studies has shown that the benefit from steroids may not be as significant as previously found. The one possible significant benefit is reduction of hearing loss in survivors, and adverse neurological outcomes.

Viral meningitis

Viral meningitis typically requires supportive therapy only; most viruses responsible for causing meningitis are not amenable to specific treatment. Viral meningitis tends to run a more benign course than bacterial meningitis. Herpes simplex virus and varicella zoster virus may respond to treatment with antiviral drugs such as acyclovir, but there are no clinical trials that have specifically addressed whether this treatment is effective. Mild cases of viral meningitis can be treated at home with conservative measures such as fluid, bedrest, and analgesics.

Fungal meningitis

Fungal meningitis, such as cryptococcal meningitis, is treated with long courses of highly dosed antifungals, such as amphotericin Band flucytosine Raised intracranial pressure is common in fungal meningitis, and frequent (ideally daily) lumbar punctures to relieve the pressure are recommended, or alternatively a lumbar drain.

prognosis

Untreated, bacterial meningitis is almost always fatal. Viral meningitis, in contrast, tends to resolve spontaneously and is rarely fatal. With treatment, mortality (risk of death) from bacterial meningitis depends on the age of the patient and the underlying cause. Of the newborn patients, 20–30% may die from an episode of bacterial meningitis. This risk is much lower in older children, whose mortality is about 2%, but rises again to about 19–37% in adults. Risk of death is predicted by various factors apart from age, such as the pathogen and the time it takes for the pathogen to be cleared from the cerebrospinal fluid, the severity of the generalized illness, decreased level of consciousness or abnormally low count of white blood cells in the CSF. Meningitis caused by *H. influenzae* and meningococci has a better prognosis compared to cases caused by group B streptococci, coliforms and *S. pneumonia*. In adults, too, meningococcal meningitis has a lower mortality (3–7%) than pneumococcal disease.

In children there are several potential disabilities which result from damage to the nervous system. Sensorineural hearing loss, epilepsy, learning and behavioral difficulties, as well as decreased intelligence, occur in about 15% of survivors. Some of the hearing loss may be reversible. In adults, 66% of all cases emerge without disability. The main problems

are deafness (in 14%) and cognitive impairment (in 10%).

CHAPTER TWENTY-EIGHT

RENAL COLIC & HYPOGLYCEMIA

Renal colic is a type of pain commonly caused by kidney stones.

The pain typically begins in the loin region and often radiates to the hypochondrium or the groin. The pain is often colicky (comes in waves) due to ureteric peristalsis, but may be constant. It may come in two varieties: dull and acute; the acute variation is particularly unpleasant and is often described as one of the strongest pain sensations felt by humans (being worse than childbirth, broken bones, gunshot wounds, burns, or surgery).

Depending on the type and size/s of the kidney stones moving through the urinal tract the pain may be stronger in the renal or bladder area or equally strong in both. In lower obstructions, males may experience pain in the genitals.

Prognosis and treatment

Most small stones are passed spontaneously and only pain management is required. Diclofenac and antispasmodics like Hyoscine butyl bromide can be used. But the doctor must not give morphine to soothe the pain, because it raises ureteral pressure, worsening the condition. There is typically no antalgic position for the patient (lying down on the non- aching side and applying a hot bottle or towel to the area affected may help). If the pain is not too intense, a speedier release of the stones may be achieved by walking. Larger stones may require surgical intervention for their removal, like percutaneous nephrolithotomy.

Hypoglycemia

Hypoglycemia or hypoglycaemia (not to be confused with hyperglycemia) is the medical term for a state produced by a lower than normal level of blood glucose. The term literally means "under-sweet blood" . It can produce a variety of symptoms and effects but the principal problems arise from an inadequate supply of glucose to the brain, resulting in impairment of function (neuroglycopenia). Effects can range from mild dysphoria to more serious issues such as seizures, unconsciousness, and (rarely) permanent brain damage or death.

The most common forms of hypoglycemia occur as a complication of treatment of diabetes mellitus with insulin or oral medications. Hypoglycemia is less common in non-diabetic persons, but can occur at any age. Among the causes are excessive insulin produced in the body (hyperinsulinemia), inborn errors of metabolism, medications and poisons, alcohol, hormone deficiencies, prolonged starvation, alterations of metabolism associated with infection, and organ failure.

Hypoglycemia is treated by restoring the blood glucose level to normal by the ingestion or administration of dextrose or carbohydrate foods. In more severe circumstances it is treated by injection or infusion of glucagon. Recurrent hypoglycemia may be prevented by reversing or removing the underlying cause, by increasing the frequency of meals, with medications like diazoxide, octreotide, or glucocorticoids, or by surgical removal of much of the pancreas.

The level of blood glucose low enough to define hypoglycemia may be different for different people, in different circumstances, and for different purposes, and occasionally has been a matter of controversy. Most healthy adults maintain fasting glucose levels above 4.0mmol/L (72 mg/dl), and develop symptoms of hypoglycemia when the glucose falls below 4 mmol/L. It can sometimes be difficult to determine whether a person's symptoms are due to hypoglycemia. Criteria referred to as Whipple's triad are used to determine a diagnosis of hypoglycemia: Symptoms known to be caused by hypoglycemia

Low glucose at the time the symptoms occur Reversal or improvement of symptoms or problems when the glucose is restored to normal

Hypoglycemia (common usage) is also a term in popular culture and alternative medicine for a common, often self-diagnosed, condition characterized by shakiness and altered mood and thinking, but without measured low glucose or risk of severe harm. It is treated by changing eating patterns.

In those treated for diabetes, a diagnosis of hypoglycemia can be made based on the presence of low blood sugar alone. Otherwise, Whipple's triad is required which include symptoms consistent with hypoglycemia, a low blood sugar, and resolution of these symptoms once the blood sugar improves.

Throughout a 24 hour period, blood plasma glucose levels are generally maintained between 4-8 mmol/L (72 and 144 mg/dL).[11] Although 3.3 or 3.9 mmol/L (60 or 70 mg/dL) is commonly cited as the lower limit of normal glucose, symptoms of hypoglycemia usually do not occur until 2.8 to 3.0 mmol/L.(50 to 54 mg/dl)

The precise level of glucose considered low enough to define hypoglycemia is dependent on (1) the measurement method, (2) the age of the person, (3) presence or absence of effects, and (4) the purpose of the definition.

Method of measurement

Blood glucose levels discussed in this article are venous plasma or serum levels measured by standard, automated glucose oxidase methods used in medical laboratories. For clinical purposes, plasma and serum levels are similar enough to be interchangeable. Arterial plasma or serum levels are slightly higher than venous levels, and capillary levels are typically in between. This difference between arterial and venous levels is small in the fasting state but is amplified and can be greater than 10% in the postprandial state. On the other hand, whole blood glucose levels (e.g., by fingerpick meters) are about 10%-15% lower than venous plasma levels. Furthermore, available fingerstick glucose meters are only warranted to be accurate to within 15% of a simultaneous laboratory value under optimal conditions and home use in the investigation of hypoglycemia is fraught with misleading low numbers. In other words, a meter glucose reading of 39 mg/dL could be properly obtained from a person whose laboratory serum glucose was 53 mg/dL; even wider variations can occur with "real world" home use.

Two other factors significantly affect glucose measurement: hematocrit and delay after blood draw. The disparity between venous and whole blood concentrations is greater when the hematocrit is high, as in newborn infants, or adults with polycythemia. High neonatal hematocrits are particularly likely to confound glucose measurement by the meter. Second, unless the specimen is drawn into a fluoride tube or processed immediately to separate the serum or plasma from the cells, the measurable glucose will be gradually lowered by *in vitro* metabolism of the glucose at a rate of approximately 7 mg/dL/hr., or even more in the presence of leukocytosis The delay that occurs when blood is drawn at a satellite site and transported to a central laboratory hours later for routine processing is a common cause of mildly low glucose levels in general chemistry panels.

Age differences

Children's blood sugar levels are often slightly lower than adults. Overnight fasting glucose levels are below 70 mg/dL (3.9 mM) in 5% of healthy adults, but up to 5% of children can be below 60 mg/dL (3.3 mM) in the morning fasting state. As the duration of fasting is extended, a higher percentage of infants and children will have mildly low plasma glucose levels, usually without symptoms. The normal range of newborn blood sugars continues to be debated. It has been proposed that newborn brains are able to use alternate fuels when glucose levels are low more readily than adults. Experts continue to debate the significance and risk of such levels, though the trend has been to recommend the maintenance of glucose levels above 60–70 mg/dL the first day after birth.

Presence or absence of effects

Research in healthy adults shows that mental efficiency declines slightly but measurably as blood glucose falls below 65 mg/dL (3.6 mM) in many people. Hormonal defense mechanisms (adrenaline and glucagon) are normally activated as it drops below a threshold level (about 55 mg/dL (3.0 mM) for most people), producing the typical hypoglycemic symptoms of shakiness and dysphoria.[1589] Obvious impairment may not occur until the glucose falls below 40 mg/dL (2.2 mM), and many healthy people may occasionally have glucose levels below 65 in the morning without apparent effects. Since the brain effects of hypoglycemia, termed neuroglycopenia, determine whether a given low glucose is a "problem" for that person, most doctors use the term *hypoglycemia* only when a moderately low glucose level is accompanied by symptoms or brain effects.

Determining the presence of both parts of this definition is not always straightforward, as hypoglycemic symptoms and effects are vague and can be produced by other conditions; people with recurrently low glucose levels can lose their threshold symptoms so that severe neuroglycopenic impairment can occur without much warning, and many measurement methods (especially glucose meters) are imprecise at low levels.

Diabetic hypoglycemia represents a special case with respect to the relationship of measured glucose and hypoglycemic symptoms for several reasons. First, although home glucose meter readings are often misleading, the probability that a low reading, whether accompanied by symptoms or not, represents real hypoglycemia is much higher in a person who takes insulin than in someone who does not. Second, because injected insulin cannot be "turned off," diabetic hypoglycemia has a greater chance of progressing to serious impairment if not treated, compared to most other forms of hypoglycemia. Third, because glucose levels are often above normal for long periods of time (hours, days, or months) in persons with diabetes, hypoglycemic symptoms may sometimes occur at higher thresholds than in people whose blood sugar is usually normal. For all of these reasons, higher meter glucose thresholds are often considered "hypoglycemic" in people with diabetes.

Signs and symptoms

Hypoglycemic symptoms and manifestations can be divided into those produced by the counterregulatory hormones (epinephrine/adrenaline and glucagon) triggered by the falling glucose, and the neuroglycopenic effects produced by the reduced brain sugar.

Adrenergic manifestations
Shakiness, anxiety, nervousness
Palpitations, tachycardia
Sweating, feeling of warmth (although sweat glands have muscarinic receptors, thus "adrenergic manifestations" is not entirely accurate)
Pallor, coldness, clamminess
Dilated pupils (mydriasis)
Feeling of numbness "pins and needles" (paresthesia)
Glucagon manifestations
Hunger, borborygmus
Nausea, vomiting, abdominal discomfort
Headache
Neuroglycopenic manifestations
Abnormal mentation, impaired judgment
Nonspecific dysphoria, moodiness, depression, crying, exaggerated concerns
Negativism, irritability, belligerence, combativeness, rage
Personality change, emotional lability
Fatigue, weakness, apathy, lethargy, daydreaming, sleep

- Confusion, amnesia, dizziness, delirium
- Staring, "glassy" look, blurred vision, double vision
- Flashes of light in the field of vision
- Automatic behavior, also known as automatism
- Difficulty speaking, slurred speech
- Ataxia, incoordination, sometimes mistaken for "drunkenness"
- Focal or general motor deficit, paralysis, hemiparesis
- Paresthesia, headache
- Stupor, coma, abnormal breathing
- Generalized or focal seizures

Not all of the above manifestations occur in every case of hypoglycemia. There is no consistent order to the appearance of the symptoms if symptoms even occur. Specific manifestations may also vary by age, by the severity of the hypoglycemia and the speed of the decline. In young children, vomiting can sometimes accompany morning hypoglycemia with ketosis. In older children and adults, moderately severe hypoglycemia can resemble mania, mental illness, drug intoxication, or drunkenness. In the elderly, hypoglycemia can produce focal stroke-like effects or a hard-to-define malaise. The symptoms of a single person may be similar from episode to episode, but are not necessarily so and may be influenced by the speed at which glucose levels are dropping, as well as previous incidence.

In newborns, hypoglycemia can produce irritability, jitters, myoclonic jerks, cyanosis, respiratory distress, apneic episodes, sweating, hypothermia, somnolence, hypotonia, refusal to feed, and seizures or "spells." Hypoglycemia can resemble asphyxia, hypocalcemia, sepsis, or heart failure.

In both young and old patients, the brain may habituate to low glucose levels, with a reduction of noticeable symptoms despite neuroglycopenic impairment. In insulin-dependent diabetic patients, this phenomenon is termed *hypoglycemia unawareness* and is a significant clinical problem when improved glycemic control is attempted. Another aspect of this phenomenon occurs in type I glycogenosis, when chronic hypoglycemia before diagnosis may be better tolerated than acute hypoglycemia after treatment is underway.

In nearly all cases, hypoglycemia that is severe enough to cause seizures or unconsciousness can be reversed without obvious harm to the brain. Cases of death or permanent neurological damage occurring with a single episode have usually involved prolonged, untreated unconsciousness, interference with breathing, severe concurrent disease, or some other type of vulnerability. Nevertheless, brain damage or death has occasionally resulted from severe hypoglycemia.

Causes

The circumstances of hypoglycemia provide most of the clues to the diagnosis. Circumstances include the age of the patient, time of day, time since last meal, previous episodes, nutritional status, physical and mental development, drugs or toxins (especially insulin or other diabetes drugs), diseases of other organ systems, family history, and response to treatment. When hypoglycemia occurs repeatedly, a record or "diary" of the spells over several months, noting the circumstances of each spell (time of day, relation to last meal, nature of last meal, response to carbohydrate, and so forth) may be useful in recognizing the nature and cause of the hypoglycemia.

An especially important aspect is whether the patient is seriously ill with another problem. Severe disease of nearly all major organ systems can cause hypoglycemia as a secondary problem. Hospitalized patients, especially in intensive care units or those prevented from eating, can suffer hypoglycemia from a variety of circumstances related to the care of their primary disease. Hypoglycemia in these circumstances is often multifactorial or even iatrogenic. Once identified, these types of hypoglycemia are readily reversed and prevented, and the underlying disease becomes the primary problem.

Apart from determining nutritional status and identifying whether there is likely to be an underlying disease more serious than hypoglycemia, the physical examination of the patient is only occasionally helpful. Macrosomia in infancy usually indicates hyperinsulinism. A few syndromes and metabolic diseases may be recognizable by clues such as hepatomegaly or macropains.

It may take longer to recover from severe hypoglycemia with unconsciousness or seizure even after the restoration of normal blood glucose. When a person has not been unconscious, failure of carbohydrate to reverse the symptoms in 10–15 minutes increases the likelihood that hypoglycemia was not the cause of the symptoms. When severe hypoglycemia has persisted in a hospitalized patient, the amount of glucose required to maintain satisfactory blood glucose levels becomes an important clue to the underlying aetiology. Glucose requirements above 10 mg/kg/minute in infants or 6 mg/kg/minute in children and adults are strong evidence for hyperinsulinism. In this context, this is referred to as the *glucose infusion rate* (GIR). Finally, the blood glucose response to glucagon given when the glucose is low can also help distinguish among various types of hypoglycemia. A rise of blood glucose by more than 30 mg/dl (1.70 mmol/l) suggests insulin excess as the probable cause of the hypoglycemia.

Newborn infants

Hypoglycemia is a common problem in critically ill or extremely low birth weight infants. If not due to maternal hyperglycemia, in most cases it is multifactorial, transient and easily supported. In a minority of cases, hypoglycemia turns out to be due to significant hyperinsulinism, hypopituitarism or an inborn error of metabolism and presents more of a management challenge.

- Transient neonatal hypoglycemia
- Prematurity, intrauterine growth retardation, perinatal asphyxia
- Maternal hyperglycemia due to diabetes or iatrogenic glucose administration
- Sepsis
- Prolonged fasting (e.g., due to inadequate breast milk or condition interfering with feeding)
- Congenital hypopituitarism
- Congenital hyperinsulinism, several types, both transient and persistent
- Inborn errors of carbohydrate metabolism such as glycogen storage disease

Young children

Single episodes of hypoglycemia may occur due to gastroenteritis or fasting, but recurrent episodes nearly always indicate either an inborn error of metabolism, congenital hypopituitarism, or congenital hyperinsulinism. A list of common causes:

- Prolonged fasting
- Diarrheal illness in young children, especially rotavirus gastroenteritis
- Idiopathic ketotic hypoglycemia
- Isolated growth hormone deficiency, hypopituitarism
- Insulin excess
- Hyperinsulinism due to several congenital disorders of insulin secretion
- Insulin injected for type 1 diabetes
  - Hyper insulin Hyper ammonia syndrome (HIHA) due to Glutamate dehydrogenase 1 gene. Can cause mental retardation and epilepsy in severe cases.
- Gastric dumping syndrome (after gastrointestinal surgery)
- Other congenital metabolic diseases; some of the common include
- Maple syrup urine disease and other organic acidurias
- Type 1 glycogen storage disease

Type III glycogen storage disease. Can cause less severe hypoglycemia than type I
Phosphoenolpyruvate carboxin's deficiency, causes metabolic acidosis and severe hypoglycemia.
Disorders of fatty acid oxidation
Medium chain acylal dehydrogenase deficiency (MCAD)
Familial Leucine sensitive hypoglycemia
Accidental ingestions
Sulfonylureas, propranolol and others
Ethanol (mouthwash, "leftover morning-after-the-party drinks")

Young adults

By far, the most common cause of severe hypoglycemia in this age range is insulin injected for type 1 diabetes. Circumstances should provide clues fairly quickly for the new diseases causing severe hypoglycemia. All of the congenital metabolic defects, congenital forms of hyperinsulinism, and congenital hypopituitarism are likely to have already been diagnosed or are unlikely to start causing new hypoglycemia at this age. Body mass is large enough to make starvation hypoglycemia and idiopathic ketotic hypoglycemia quite uncommon.

Recurrent mild hypoglycemia may fit a reactive hypoglycemia pattern, but this is also the peak age for idiopathic postprandial syndrome, and recurrent "spells" in this age group can be traced to orthostatic hypotension or hyperventilation as often as demonstrable hypoglycemia.

Insulin-induced hypoglycemia
Insulin injected for type 1 diabetes
Factitious insulin injection (Munchausen syndrome)
Insulin-secreting pancreatic tumor
Reactive hypoglycemia and idiopathic postprandial syndrome
Addison's disease
Sepsis

Older adults

The incidence of hypoglycemia due to complex drug interactions, especially involving oral hypoglycemic agents and insulin for diabetes, rises with age. Though much rarer, the incidence of insulin-producing tumors also rises with advancing age. Most tumors causing hypoglycemia by mechanisms other than insulin excess occur in adults.

Insulin-induced hypoglycemia
Insulin injected for diabetes
Factitious insulin injection (Munchausen syndrome)
Excessive effects of oral diabetes drugs, beta-blockers, or drug interactions
Insulin-secreting pancreatic tumor
Alcohol induced hypoglycemia often linked with ketoacidosis (depletion of NAD+ leads to a block of gluconeogenesis)
Alimentary (rapid jejunal emptying with exaggerated insulin response)
After gastrectomy dumping syndrome or bowel bypass surgery or resection
Reactive hypoglycemia and idiopathic postprandial syndrome
Tumor hypoglycemia, Doege-Potter syndrome
Acquired adrenal insufficiency
Acquired hypopituitarism
Immunopathologic hypoglycemia

Pathophysiology of Hypoglycemia

Like most animal tissues, brain metabolism depends primarily on glucose for fuel in most circumstances. A limited amount of glucose can be derived from glycogen stored in astrocytes, but it is consumed within minutes. For most practical purposes, the brain is dependent on a continual supply of glucose diffusing from the blood into the interstitial tissue within the central nervous system and into the neurons themselves.

Therefore, if the amount of glucose supplied by the blood falls, the brain is one of the first organs affected. In most people, a subtle reduction of mental efficiency can be observed when the glucose falls below 65 mg/dl (3.6 mM). Impairment of action and judgment usually becomes obvious below 40 mg/dl (2.2 mM). Seizures may occur as the glucose falls further. As blood glucose levels fall below 10 mg/dl (0.55 mM), most neurons become electrically silent and nonfunctional, resulting in coma. These brain effects are collectively referred to as neuroglycopenia.

The importance of an adequate supply of glucose to the brain is apparent from the number of nervous, hormonal and metabolic responses to a falling glucose level. Most of these are defensive or adaptive, tending to raise the blood sugar via glycogenolysis and gluconeogenesis or provide alternative fuels. If the blood sugar level falls too low the liver converts a storage of glycogen into glucose and releases it into the bloodstream, to prevent the person going into a diabetic coma, for a short period of time.

Brief or mild hypoglycemia produces no lasting effects on the brain, though it can temporarily alter brain responses to additional hypoglycemia. Prolonged, severe hypoglycemia can produce lasting damage to a wide range. This can include impairment of cognitive function, motor control, or even consciousness. The likelihood of permanent brain damage from any given instance of severe hypoglycemia is difficult to estimate and depends on a multitude of factors such as age, recent blood and brain glucose experience, concurrent problems such as hypoxia, and availability of alternative fuels. It has been frequently found that those Type 1 diabetics found "dead in bed" in the morning after suspected severe hypoglycemia had some underlying coronary pathology that led to an induced fatal heart attack. Recently, several of these individuals found "dead in bed" were wearing Continuous Glucose Monitors, which provided a history of glucose levels prior to the fatal event. It has been found in several cases, that the fatal event was preceded by at least two hours of blood glucose levels under 40 mg/dl, possibly lower as the continuous glucose monitors are not accurate at levels below 40 mg/dl. The individuals failed to respond to the audible alarms produced by the continuous glucose monitor which may have been "alarming" for many hours prior to the fatal event. The vast majority of symptomatic hypoglycemic episodes result in no detectable permanent harm.

Diagnosis

When suspected hypoglycemia recurs and a critical specimen has not been obtained, the diagnostic evaluation may take several paths. However good nutrition and prompt intake are essential.

When general health is good, the symptoms are not severe, and the person can fast normally through the night, experimentation with diet (extra snacks with fat or protein, reduced sugar) may be enough to solve the problem. If it is uncertain whether "spells" are indeed due to hypoglycemia, some physicians will recommend use of a home glucose meter to test at the time of the spells to confirm that glucose are low. This approach may be most useful when spells are fairly frequent or the patient is confident that he or she can provoke a spell. The principal drawback of this approach is the high rate of false-positive or equivocal levels due to the imprecision of the currently available meters: both physician and patient need an accurate understanding of what a meter can and cannot do to avoid frustrating and inconclusive results.

In cases of recurrent hypoglycemia with severe symptoms, the best method of excluding dangerous conditions is often a *diagnostic fast*. This is usually conducted in the hospital, and the duration depends on the age of the patient and response to the fast. A healthy adult can usually maintain a glucose level above 50 mg/dl (2.8 mM) for 72 hours, a child for 36 hours, and an infant for 24 hours. The purpose of the fast is to determine whether the person can maintain his or her blood glucose as long as normal, and can respond to fasting with the appropriate metabolic changes. At the end of the fast, the insulin should be nearly undetectable and ketosis should be fully established. The patient's blood glucose levels are monitored and a critical specimen is obtained if the glucose falls. Despite its unpleasantness and expense, a diagnostic fast may be the only effective way to confirm or refute a number of serious forms of hypoglycemia, especially those involving excessive insulin.

A traditional method for investigating suspected hypoglycemia is the oral glucose tolerance test, especially when prolonged to 3, 4, or 5 hours. Although quite popular in the United States in the 1960s, repeated research studies have demonstrated that many healthy people will have glucose levels below 70 or 60 during a prolonged test and that many types of significant hypoglycemia may go undetected with it. This combination of poor sensitivity and specificity have resulted in its abandonment for this purpose by physicians experienced in disorders of glucose metabolism.

Prevention

The most effective means of preventing further episodes of hypoglycemia depends on the cause. The risk of further episodes of diabetic hypoglycemia can often (but not always) be reduced by lowering the dose of insulin or other medications, or by more meticulous attention to blood sugar balance during unusual hours, higher levels of exercise, or alcohol intake.

Many of the inborn errors of metabolism require avoidance or shortening of fasting intervals or extra carbohydrates. For the more severe disorders, such as type 1 glycogen storage disease, this may be supplied in the form of cornstarch every few hours or by continuous gastric infusion.

Several treatments are used for hyperinsulinemia hypoglycemia, depending on the exact form and severity. Some forms of congenital hyperinsulinism respond to diazoxide or octreotide. Surgical removal of the overactive part of the pancreas is curative with minimal risk when hyperinsulinism is focal or due to a benign insulin-producing tumor of the pancreas. When congenital hyperinsulinism is diffuse and refractory to medications, near-total pancreatectomy may be the treatment of last resort, but in this condition is less consistently effective and fraught with more complications.

Hypoglycemia due to hormone deficiencies such as hypopituitarism or adrenal insufficiency usually ceases when the appropriate hormone is replaced.

Hypoglycemia due to dumping syndrome and other post-surgical conditions is best dealt with by altering diet. Including fat and protein with carbohydrates may slow digestion and reduce early insulin secretion. Some forms of this respond to treatment with a glucosidase inhibitor, which slows starch digestion.

Reactive hypoglycemia with demonstrably low blood glucose levels is most often a predictable nuisance which can be avoided by consuming fat and protein with carbohydrates, by adding morning or afternoon snacks, and reducing alcohol intake.

Idiopathic postprandial syndrome without demonstrably low glucose levels at the time of symptoms can be more of a management challenge. Many people find improvement by changing eating patterns (smaller meals, avoiding excessive sugar, mixed meals rather than carbohydrates by themselves), reducing intake of stimulants such as caffeine, or by making lifestyle changes to reduce stress. See the following section of this article.

Treatment

Management of hypoglycemia involves immediately raising the blood sugar to normal, determining the cause, and taking measures to hopefully prevent future episodes.

The blood glucose can be raised to normal within minutes by taking (or receiving) 10-

20 grams of carbohydrate. It can be taken as food or drink if the person is conscious and able to swallow. This amount of carbohydrate is contained in about 3-4 ounces (100-120 ml) of orange, apple, or grape juice although fruit juices contain a higher proportion of fructose which is more slowly metabolized than pure dextrose, alternatively, about 4-5 ounces (120- 150 ml) of regular (non-diet) soda may also work, as will about one slice of bread, about 4 crackers, or about 1 serving of most starchy foods. Starch is quickly digested to glucose (unless the person is taking acarbose), but adding fat or protein retards digestion.

Symptoms should begin to improve within 5 minutes, though full recovery may take 10–20 minutes. Overfeeding does not speed recovery and if the person has diabetes will simply produce hyperglycemia afterwards.

If a person is suffering such severe effects of hypoglycemia that they cannot (due to combativeness) or should not (due to seizures or unconsciousness) be given anything by mouth, medical personnel such as EMTs and paramedics, or in-hospital personnel can establish an IV and give intravenous dextrose, concentrations varying depending on age (infants are given 2 ml/kg dextrose 10%, children are given dextrose 25%, and adults are given dextrose 50%). Care must be taken in giving these solutions because they can be very necrotic if the IV is infiltrated. If an IV cannot be established, the patient can be given 1 to 2 milligrams of glucagon in an intramuscular injection. More treatment information can be found in the article diabetic hypoglycemia.

One situation where starch may be less effective than glucose or sucrose is when a person is taking acarbose. Since acarbose and other alpha-glucosidase inhibitors prevents starch and other sugars from being broken down into monosaccharides that can be absorbed by the body, patients taking these medications should consume monosaccharide-containing foods such as glucose tablets, honey, or juice to reverse hypoglycemia.

CHAPTER TWENTY-NINE

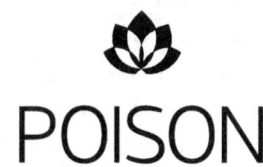

POISON

In the context of biology, poisons are substances that can cause disturbances to organisms, usuallyby chemical reaction or other activity on the molecular scale, when a sufficient quantity is absorbed by an organism. In medicine (particularly veterinary) and in zoology, a poison is often distinguished from a toxin and a venom. Toxins are poisons produced via some biological function in nature, and venoms are usually defined as biological toxins that are injected by a bite or sting to cause their effect, while other poisons are genera lly defined as substances which are absorbed through epithelial linings such as the skin or gut.

Some poisons are also toxins, usually referring to naturally produced substances, such as the bacterial proteins that cause tetanus and botulism. A distinction between the two terms is not always observed, even among scientists.

Animal toxins that are delivered subcutaneously (e.g. by sting or bite) are also called *venom*. In normal usage, a poisonous organism is one that is harmful to consume, but a venomous organism uses poison to defend itself while still alive. A single organism can be both venomous and poisonous.

The derivative forms "toxic" and "poisonous" are synonymous.In nuclear physics, a poison is a substance that obstructs or inhibits a nuclear reaction. For an example, see nuclear poison.

Paracelsus, the father of toxicology, once wrote: "Everything is poison, there is poison in everything. Only the dose makes a thing not a poison." The term "poison" is often used colloquially to describe any harmful substance, particularly corrosive substances, carcinogens, mutagens, teratogens and harmful pollutants, and to exaggerate the dangers of chemicals. The legal definition of "poison" is stricter. A medical condition of poisoning can also be caused by substances that are not legally required to carry the label "poison".

Environmentally hazardous substances are not necessarily poisoning and vice versa. For example, food industry wastewater - which may contain milk or potato juice - can be hazardous to the ecosystems of streams and rivers by consuming oxygen and causing eutrophication, but is nonhazardous to humans and not classified as a poison.

Uses of poison

Throughout human history, intentional application of poison has been used as a method Of assassination, murder, suicide, and execution. As a method of execution, poison has been ingested, as the ancient Athenians did (see Socrates), inhaled, as with carbon monoxide or hydrogen cyanide (see gas chamber), or injected (see lethal injection). Many languages describe lethal injection with their corresponding words for "poison shot". Poison's lethal effect can be combined with its allegedly magical powers; an example is the Chinese *gu* poison. Poison was also employed in gunpowder warfare.

The term poison with regards to biology and chemistry is often misused due to lack of a universal definition. Biologically speaking, any substance if given in large enough amounts is poisonous and can cause death. For instance, while botulinum toxin is lethal on the level of nanograms, a person would have to ingest kilograms worth of water to receive a lethal dose.

Biological poisoning

Acute poisoning is exposure to a poison on one occasion or during a short period of time. Symptoms develop in close relation to the exposure. Absorption of a poison is necessary for systemic poisoning. In contrast, substances that destroy tissue but do not absorb, such as lye, are classified as corrosives rather than poisons. Furthermore, many common household medications are not labeled with skull and crossbones, although they can cause severe illness or even death. In the medical sense, poisoning can be caused by less dangerous substances than those receiving the legal classification of "poison".

Chronic poisoning is long-term repeated or continuous exposure to a poison where symptoms do not occur immediately or after each exposure. The patient gradually becomes ill, or becomes ill after a long latent period.

Chronic poisoning most commonly occurs following exposure to poisons that bioaccumulate, or are biomagnified, such as mercury and lead.

Contact or absorption of poisons can cause rapid death or impairment. Agents that act on the nervous system can paralyze in seconds or less, and include both biologically derived neurotoxins and so-called nerve gases, which may be synthesized for warfare or industry.

Inhaled or ingested cyanide, used as a method of execution in gas chambers, almost instantly starves the body of energy by inhibiting the enzymes in mitochondria that make ATP. Intravenous injection of an unnaturally high concentration of potassium chloride, such as in the execution of prisoners in parts of the United States, quickly stops the heart by eliminating the cell potential necessary for muscle contraction.

Most biocides, including pesticides, are created to act as poisons to target organisms, although acute or less observable chronic poisoning can also occur in non-target organism, including the humans who apply the biocides and other beneficial organisms. For example, the herbicide 2,4-D imitates the action of a plant hormone, to the effect that the lethal toxicity is specific to plants. Indeed, 2,4 -D is not a poison, but classified as "harmful" (EU).

The study of the symptoms, mechanisms, treatment and diagnosis of biological poisoning is known as toxicology.

Initial management

Initial management for all poisonings includes ensuring adequate cardiopulmonary function and providing treatment for any symptoms such as seizures, shock, and pain.

Poisons that have been injected (e.g. from the sting of poisonous animals) can be treated by binding the affected body part with a pressure bandage and by placing the affected body part in hot water (with a temperature of 50°C). The pressure bandage makes sure the poison is not pumped throughout the body and the hot water breaks down the poison. This treatment however only works with poisons that are composed of protein-molecules.

Decontamination

If the toxin was recently ingested, absorption of the substance may be able to be decreased through gastric decontamination. This may be achieved using activated charcoal, gastric lavage, whole bowel irrigation, or nasogastric aspiration. Routine use of emetics (syrup of Ipecac), cathartics or laxatives are no longer recommended.

Activated charcoal is the treatment of choice to prevent absorption of the poison. It is usually administered when the patient is in the emergency room or by a trained emergency healthcare provider such as a Paramedic or EMT. However, charcoal is ineffective against metals such as sodium, potassium, and lithium, and alcohols and glycols; it is also not recommended for ingestion of corrosive chemicals such as acids and alkalis.

Whole bowel irrigation cleanses the bowel, this is achieved by giving the patient large amounts of a polyethylene glycol solution. The osmotically balanced polyethene glycol solution is not absorbed into the body, having the effect of flushing out the entire gastrointestinal tract. Its major uses are following ingestion of sustained-release drugs, toxins that are not absorbed by activated charcoal (i.e. lithium, iron), and for the removal of ingested packets of drugs (body packing/smuggling).

Gastric lavage, commonly known as a stomach pump, is the insertion of a tube into the stomach, followed by administration of water or saline down the tube. The liquid is then removed along with the contents of the stomach. Lavage has been used for many years as a common treatment for poisoned patients. However, a recent review of the procedure in poisonings suggests no benefit. It is still sometimes used if it can be performed within 1 hour of ingestion and the exposure is potentially life-threatening.

Nasogastric aspiration involves the placement of a tube via the nose down into the stomach, the stomach contents are then removed via suction. This procedure is mainly used for liquid ingestions where activated charcoal is ineffective, e.g. ethylene glycol poisoning.

Emesis (i.e. induced by ipecac) is no longer recommended in poisoning situations, because vomiting is ineffective at removing poisons. Cathartics were postulated to decrease absorption by increasing the expulsion of the poison from the gastrointestinal tract. There are two types of cathartics used in poisoned patients; saline cathartics (sodium sulfate, magnesium citrate, magnesium sulfate) and saccharide cathartics (sorbitol). They do not appear to improve patient outcome and are no longer recommended.

Antidotes

Some poisons have specific antidotes:
> Poison/Drug
> Antidote
> paracetamol (acetaminophen)
> N-acetylcysteine
> vitamin K anticoagulants, e.g. warfarin
> vitamin K
> opioids
> Naloxone
> Iron (and other heavy metals)
> deferoxamine, Deferasirox or Deferiprone
> Benzodiazepines
> Flumazenil
> ethylene glycol
> ethanol or fomepizole, and thiamine
> Methanol
> ethanol or fomepizole, and folinic acid
> Cyanide

In some situations, elimination of the poison can be enhanced using diuresis, hemodialysis, hemoperfusion, hyperbaric medicine, peritoneal dialysis, exchange transfusion or chelation. However, this may actually worsen the poisoning in some cases, so it should always be verified based on what substances are involved.

Further treatment

In the majority of poisonings, the mainstay of management is providing supportive care for the patient,
> i.e. treating the symptoms rather than the poison.

Thank you so much, readers .

www.ingramcontent.com/pod-product-compliance
Lightning Source LLC
Chambersburg PA
CBHW081428220526
45466CB00008B/2311